Things a
Woman
Should Know
About
Style

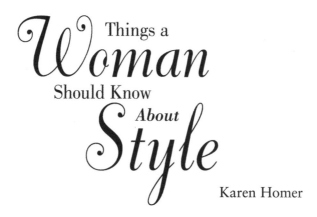

Things a Woman Should Know About Style

Karen Homer

PRION

First published in 2005.

This edition published in 2011 by
Prion
an imprint of the
Carlton Publishing Group
20 Mortimer Street
London W1T 3JW

20 19 18

Text copyright © Karen Homer 2005
Design copyright © Carlton Publishing Group

ISBN 978-1-85375-831-7

A catalogue record of this book is available from the British Library

Printed and bound in China

For Howard

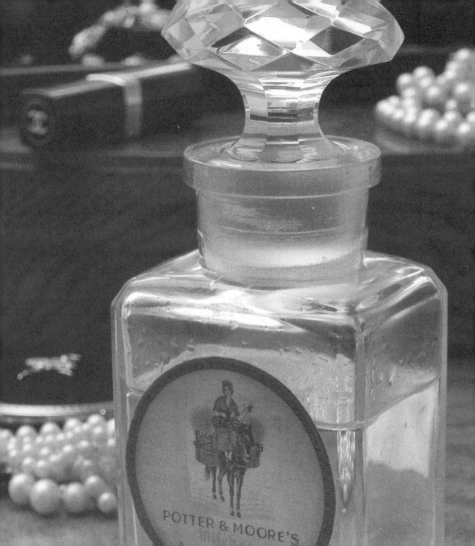

POTTER & MOORE'S

Contents

Introduction

Some people are born stylish, some people achieve style, but no one can have style thrust upon them... it comes from within.

As Coco Chanel once said, 'Fashion fades, only style remains the same,' but how do you get a sense of style? It can't be bought, no matter how much you spend, as many a Hollywood actress has learnt the hard way, caught by the paparazzi in another too-revealing designer dress. Nor can you employ someone to find it for you. One look at the clothes so-called celebrity stylists wear themselves is enough to confirm that blind trust in another person's sense of style is a mistake.

The good news is that style can be developed. It's not easy to be a twenty-first-century style icon. We don't have the fashion uniform our mothers and grandmothers enjoyed – or hated. There's so much choice today that's it's all too easy to get it wrong and there's always someone out there ready to laugh at our fashion faux pas. But if you're happy to take on board a few hard and fast rules, some constructive criticism and the occasional shout of protest, then this book can help you dis-cover some rules of classic style that will never let you down. I'm not saying that boob tubes are a bad idea …but they are.

What follows is a book about STYLE – classic, timeless style. You may not achieve it every day; you may not even want it every day, but if you're interested in pulling off an Audrey Hepburn or a Grace Kelly, this is the way to do it.

So prepare to learn some insider tips – have you ever won-dered how those see-through film-premiere dresses stay on or asked exactly what is a Hollywood wax? Follow the rules and you might find yourself better prepared for situations and

Things a Woman Should Know About Style

'Vain trifles as they seem, clothes... change our view of the world and the world's view of us.'

— Virginia Woolf

environments that still do have a dress code. At the very least, with your new sartorial vocabulary you will sound like you know what you are talking about, even if the style icon within you remains resolutely buried beneath layers of spandex.

You don't have to follow fashion to know that appearance counts. Ask a politician's wife. Cherie Blair may never live down a style blunder such as answering the door to the press in her nightie. Fortunately for the rest of us, dressing impeccably all the time isn't so important.

When to care about what you wear: first dates, interviews, photographs that may be seen by your ex-husband's new wife.

When not to care about what you wear: in bed (unless on a first date), in the gym, family photographs for your mum to display on the mantlepiece, which by definition must involve sartorial horrors.

If psychologists are to be believed, dressing well can get you a better job, better friends, better sex and higher self-esteem. Do you need another excuse to go shopping?

Dressing well is like kissing: fun, but you have to practise a lot before you get it right.

Once you've got it right, you'll never lose it.

'Fashion fades, only style remains the same.'

— Coco Chanel

Gabrielle 'Coco' Chanel was truly an icon of our times. Described by George Bernard Shaw as one of the two most important women living in the world (the other being Marie Curie), she knew her worth. One of the most famous stories is of her response to the Duke of Westminster's proposal of marriage. Turning him down, Chanel said, 'There have been many Duchesses of Westminster, but there is only one "Coco" Chanel.'

It was Chanel's own style, introducing masculine elements in a truly feminine way, that gave truth to this remark. Her defiant use of trousers and traditional tailoring to give women the same kind of practical yet stylish clothes that men took for granted set a style standard for many generations of women. Anyone looking for a blueprint for easy elegance could do worse than to take a leaf out of Chanel's design book. Even today there are few outfits more stylish than the trademark tailored suit or the relaxed pleat-fronted trousers and fine jersey sweater so beloved of Coco herself.

There is a fundamental difference between style and fashion: longevity. It is far better to create for yourself a sense of style that will endure than try to keep up with the vaguaries of fashion. The tricks of classic style are timeless, and so should your clothes be if you tread carefully around the temptations of high fashion. By high fashion I mean this season's hottest designer whose wisp of a slip dress will cost you the earth and only comes in a size six. Please, get real.

There are plenty of women who will put their name on a waiting list for this dress. The woman who is trying to find her own sense of classic style is not one of them. To buy into the world of high fashion you need a virtually

'Fashions are like human beings. They come in, nobody knows when, why, or how, and they go out, nobody knows when, why, or how.'

— Charles Dickens

limitless disposable income. Or a husband with a seven-figure salary whose credit card you spend more time with than with him.

Alternatively you need to be happy buying a lot of cheap clothes.

Cheap copies of high-fashion clothes can look good, but only if you are sixteen years old. If you are over thirty and less than physically perfect, cheap clothes look cheap. Only the young and beautiful and unscrupulous advertising folk can get away with calling cheap clothes 'inexpensive'. For perfect mortals they are a bargain way to wear this season's look. For you, alas, they are a waste of money.

Far better to distance yourself from the grasping, 'must have the latest such-and-such' mentality and adopt an attitude of aloofness. You don't need to follow fashion's whims, because you have a sense of style. Better still to realise the effect on your bank balance when you stop buying clothes you hardly wear.

For a real awakening, look in your wardrobe and see how many clothes you absolutely had to have that are now stuffed to the back unworn. And yes, they do still count if you bought them in the sales.

So you'll be better off and you'll look good too. Consistently good as opposed to the occasional lucky strike when something that actually suits you comes into fashion.

'Fashion makes fools of some, sinners of others and slaves of all.'

— Josh Billings, nineteenth-century commentator

When Style Went Out of Fashion

Fashion and style happily coincided under the guidance of Chanel in the 1920s and '30s, and even under the pressures of war shortages in the 1940s women bought Norman Hartnell's utility dresses: style on a ration coupon. 1947 brought the flamboyant New Look, pioneered by Christian Dior and woven into the establishment through Hardy Amies' designs for the princesses Elizabeth and Margaret.

From the 1960s, changing moral attitudes and the sexual revolution sent skirts sky-rocketing to the tops of women's thighs.

Later hippy chic blurred the distinction between the sexes almost completely with flower power and long hair for men and women alike.

In the 1970s social unrest, high unemployment and the women's movement made fashion a target for political attack. Punk in the mid '70s, Malcolm MacLaren's Sex Pistols and Vivienne Westwood embodied the emergence of street fashion, the perfect antidote for a public tired of hippy naturalism.

In the 1980s a new glamour in the form of power dressing from Italian designers and the influence of shoulder-pad-toting soap stars in *Dallas* and *Dynasty* led to a vogue for ostentatious – and vulgar – displays of wealth. Fur, leather and gold featured prominently in the collections of designers such as Versace and Armani. Mixed up in all the sharp suits were the New Romantics – a softer, retro fashion statement harking back to hippy lace, flounce and men in make-up.

Things a Woman Should Know About Style

> *'The economic logic of fashion depends on making the old-fashioned look absurd.'*

— John Berger

By the 1990s the current fashion designer's trick of looking backwards for inspiration had firmly asserted itself. Designers like Romeo Gigli were re-inventing a softer classicism and turning the street trend for retro and vintage dressing into a profitable marketing ploy. Style, they had realised, was a thing of the past.

Fashion designers may take inspiration from the fashions of previous decades, but it is no accident that when designers proclaim an '80s comeback, the clothes you dig out that you actually wore in the 1980s look as terrible as you remember. A subtle design twist, the use of some contemporary fabric and a hefty price tag are all it requires to make a garment ''80sinspired', cleverly leaving your old clothes still horribly out-moded. How would designers stay in business otherwise?

Nevertheless, it is alarming how fashion can brainwash us, making sartorial crimes of yesteryear seem like the next big thing. Before we are tempted to revisit drainpipe jeans and ruched-top boots, it is good to remind ourselves of some horrors that have plagued our wardrobes through the decades. Still feel like buying that '70s-style peasant smock?

The Worst of...

The 1960s: The pelmet, sworn enemy of girls with cellulite; Mods and Rockers in green parka anoraks; false eyelashes that fell off into your cocktail; Bunny girls.

The 1970s: Cropped, bell-bottomed tartan trousers *à la* Bay City Rollers; the Victorian Dolly look – lace petticoats and pirate skirts; hippie's dreamy cheesecloth shirts and flares vs.

Things a Woman Should Know About Style

Punk's body piercing, bum-flaps and Nazi nick-nacks; flower power and Afghan coats that made you smell like a camel.

The 1980s: Stone-washed denim, ra-ra skirts and drainpipe trousers that flattered no one; suits with inverted-triangle jackets that made you look like an American Football player; teeny-tiny miniskirts and the constant laddering of 10-denier tights such leg-exposure caused; Big Hair and blue eyeshadow.

'Judging from the ugly and repugnant things that are sometimes in vogue, it would seem as though fashion were desirous of exhibiting its power by getting us to adopt the most atrocious things for its sake alone.'

— George Simnel, late 19th century

- Retro clothes are not stylish. Not even when you call them vintage.

- Vintage is a word used by second-hand clothes merchants to justify charging you at least ten times what the garment originally cost.

- Vintage is to adults as retro is to teenagers, it is therefore automatically more expensive.

- There are fewer and fewer genuine articles of vintage clothing around; most have been bought up by dealers, designers and film costume designers.

- There are almost no genuine vintage bargains any more. Traders have wised up.

- Any vintage clothes that still seem cheap are likely to smell of mould and fall apart as soon as you put them on. Clothes need to be cared for, not stuffed into a suitcase and stored in a damp attic for fifty years.

Things a Woman Should Know About Style

- Few people can genuinely get away with wearing vintage clothes. Clothes that may have been the epitome of style in their day just don't fit in the modern world, in more ways than one. Think about it: in the 1940s the average woman was four inches shorter and two dress sizes smaller than she is today.

- Forget vintage shoes if your feet are a size four or above.

- ...Forget vintage shoes if you are squeamish about feet.

Shoes are the one item you should never buy second hand. A shoe moulds itself to the shape of the foot of its wearer. And if even our own two feet are different in shape and size there is little chance of finding a shoe-shape match in someone else's.

Stepping Out

Shoes inspire strong feelings in women. Ask anyone who has ever drooled over a pair of four-inch satin Manolos, bought shocking pink sandals after a bad break up or has a shoe collection that runs into treble figures. So how better to start a guide to style than from the bottom up?

'Give a girl the right shoes and she can conquer the world.'

— Bette Midler

Things a Woman Should Know About Style

There are few things that can truly make or break an outfit but a pair of shoes is one of them. If you can judge a man by the state of his shoes, you can certainly size up a woman's style by what she's got on her feet.

Wearing the right shoes is imperative. You will know this if you have ever worn the wrong ones. Comfy old loafers may seem like a good idea when you have to walk to the tube, but not when you arrive at a smart dinner where everyone else is in heels. You'll feel like you did on your first day at a new school when you're in a regulation-length skirt but everyone else is in minis.

Sometimes comfort is worth sacrificing for style. But not always.

Never, ever think you can get away with cheap shoes. You can cheat with most other things, but cheap shoes look, well, cheap. Cheap leather looks like plastic. It cracks and splits rather than gently softening with wear. The soles will fall off, the uppers are probably glued, not even machine-stitched, so will start peeling away and the lack of give as you wear them will ruin your feet.

There is no need to justify expensive, classic shoes. In the long run, cheap shoes work out more expensive as they won't last you more than a year. A top-quality leather pair, on the other hand, will last for many years, with the odd re-shodding along the way. Two hundred pound black satin high-heeled court shoes are classics. Two hundred pound neon-glow patent sandals are not. And don't try to pretend they'll be 'design classics' one day.

If you spend a lot of money on a pair of shoes, Scotchguard them first and please invest in some shoe trees, and some shoe racks. Piles of shoes thrown into a wardrobe are a sorry sight, and finding a pair is impossible. Serious shoe fetishists have been known to photograph shoes and stick the picture to the outside of the shoebox. Suggestive of a control complex but not altogether a stupid idea if you have hundreds of pairs.

Things a Woman Should Know About Style

'I don't know who invented the high heel, but all women owe him a lot.'

— Marilyn Monroe

A Few More Things to Bear in Mind:
Round-toed, pointy-toed, square-toed or open-toed, they all have their place, but there are only two kinds of heels worth taking seriously: very high, or very low.

Even in the '70s platform heels were ugly, and big, wide, block heels are ugly full stop. Particularly when worn with a teeny-tiny slip dress in the style of teenage club-goers when they will be scuffed and puddle-splattered from waiting at the bus-stop for the night bus home.

Small, elegant block heels, on the other hand, are classically chic in a Jackie-Kennedy-on-campaign-trail kind of way.

The High Life

High heels have been around since the 1600s but the stiletto didn't make its debut until 1953 with the introduction of a metal spigot and moulded plastic heel. They were banned from many buildings because of the damage they caused to floors. Stilettos cause even more damage to floors since the vogue for wood and laminate flooring. Definitely wear stilettos when dining at your arch-rival's newly floored house.

Marilyn Monroe claimed to have achieved her signature hip-wiggling walk by sawing off a bit of the stiletto heel on one of each pair.

The most popular height for stiletto heels is between four and four and a half inches.

If you can't walk in stilettos, take taxis.

Things a Woman Should Know About Style

> *'It is the flagrant lack of practicality that makes high-heeled shoes so fascinating.'*

— Stephen Bayley

High-heels change your posture, therefore change the way you walk, therefore change the way you feel.

Couture-made four-inch heels are as easy to walk in as a pair of slippers. Honestly. It is not the height of the shoe that makes it easy or difficult to walk in, it is the shape.

Before you give up completely, practice tipping your weight back onto the heel of the shoe. High-heel agony comes from balancing on the ball of your foot. It will feel like you are about to do a back-flip at first, but you soon get used to it.

If you really can't learn to walk in stilettos choose heels that are wide at the top, and taper to a narrow half-inch square at the bottom.

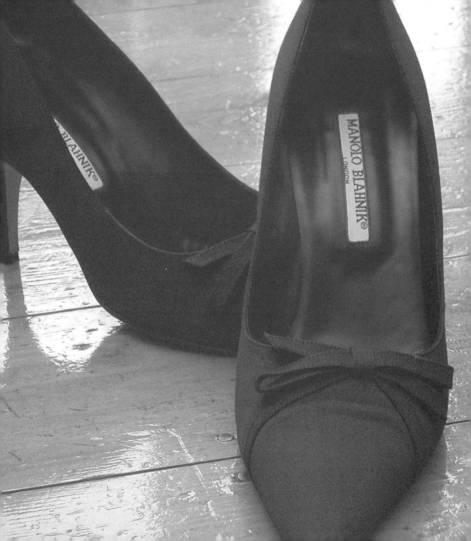

Things a Woman Should Know About Style

The highest heel that one can walk in (aside from certain fetish shoemakers, and I presume that walking is the last thing you'd do in these) is five and a half inches. The six-inch heel is a myth.

Be practical – wear pumps to work and heels to party.

If you never wear high-heeled shoes, you'll never experience the bliss that is taking them off when you get home.

Pointy shoes make your feet look narrower, but don't buy them too small or your feet will start moulding the leather around your toes. Better your feet look long, than your shoes look like bubble wrap plastic.

Plain black patent loafers are smart, comfortable and elegant: good when you wear them with evening suits, even better when you wear them with jeans. Wear them with dresses or skirts, however, and you'll look all together too Home Counties.

Round-toed ballet slippers are very chic and Audrey Hepburn, but only really suit slim ankles and small, dainty feet. Two-toned ballet slippers are a trademark Chanel look, but be careful the rest of your outfit doesn't run to gaudy – suit too pink, accessories too gold, hair too big and blond – or you will lose the chic these shoes can have. You do not want a look that needs a facelift and a Chihuahua to accessorise it.

Red shoes are the stuff of fairytale and fantasy. They exist outside the golden rule that classic style means playing it safe.

Women have a relationship with shoes that men will never understand.

Men have a relationship with women's shoes that women are better off not understanding. Never let a man drink champagne out of your shoes. Unless he buys you a new pair afterwards. Humiliate the drunken man who thinks he can drink champagne out of your strappy, open-toed sandals with a simple lesson in physics.

Things a Woman Should Know About Style

'Mama always said there's an awful lot you can tell about a person by their shoes: where they're going, where they've been.'

— Forrest Gump

Shoes can be dangerous in more ways than one: Manolo Blahnik withdrew his steel-spike stilettos from sale after being warned they could pass as a lethal weapon.

You can get away with a plain black high-street dress, as long as you are wearing a pair of fantastic shoes to go with it. This may mean that your shoes cost more than the rest of your outfit put together. That's ok.

Feel free to shoe your children in Clarks for as long as possible. Not only will they not ruin their feet, their aesthetic sensibilities will be so sharpened by years of humiliation over their wide sandals that they will never buy a nasty pair of shoes again. Memories of parties of life-or-death importance aged 13 and being forced to wear Clarke's version of the Birkenstock (about the only un-stylish thing that wasn't cool in the 1980s) still rankle.

Birkenstocks are not stylish now, nor have they ever been. If they ever become a benchmark of style it's time to give up trying.

Trained Not To

There is one kind of shoe that the style classicist can never get away with wearing. No matter how tempted you may be after a night of dancing on the balls of your feet, RESIST putting on a pair of trainers if you want to exude an aura of elegance. Trainers are not and never will be elegant, particularly if they have flashing orange stripes or brand-plugging ticks plastered all over them. The trainer may be a ubiquitous and egalitarian form of footwear, but it is best left to the purpose for which it was intended: sport. Wear your trainers to the gym.

As Manolo Blahnik once pointed out, you would never wear a swimming costume on the street so why would you wear trainers? They are, according to the king of sole couture, vulgar. And to add insult to injury, thanks to clever advertising campaigns, targeted at cool-conscious teenagers they are now horribly expensive. Teenagers will always wear trainers – you don't need to.

When you are next tempted to hang on to your youth by buying a pair of over-sized blue and silver trainers in shimmering nylon, resist. As any child will tell you, a parent in gleaming new trainers is not cool.

Never, ever buy trainers with no backs. They are entirely purposeless and ugly with it. The plain, delicate white pump, on the other hand, can look very chic in an Italian film stars tripping off gondolas wearing capri pants and pumps, bouffant hair wrapped in a chiffon scarf – kind of a way.

The worst style crime of all is wearing trainers with a suit or dress with the intention of changing into heels when you get there. Not only does it look naff it is inextricably linked to the '80s thanks to Melanie Griffiths in *Working Girl*. Plus who do you know who's got a handbag with enough spare room for another pair of shoes?

No Logo

Like the trainer, sportswear has become a class-transcending, global clothing phenomenon. Like the trainer, the shell suit is not memorable for its style. It is one of fashion's great ironies that the tracksuit is most often found cladding a physique that is less than athletic. But then fashion is full of ironies: the dry-clean only mackintosh, for example.

Don't wear logo sportswear unless you are a professional athlete and being paid for it. By logo we're talking six inch letters emblazoned across your chest, up the leg of your track pants or across the peak of your (God forbid) baseball cap. Small, discreet emblems are passable.

In fact, don't ever wear any kind of slogan emblazoned across your chest. Wit should be heard from your mouth not read off your breasts.

Especially don't wear logo sportswear if the name of the brand is just another designer label, and nothing to do with sport. This is open admission that you don't intend to raise a sweat in your gear.

When playing sport, forget about what you look like. You're in it to feel good not look good. There are times when style really isn't all that important. Cycling to work is another. Safety first: wear that cycle helmet. Even if you do look and feel ridiculous.

An exception to forgetting what you look like when indulging in sport should be made at country house parties when you are hoping to seduce your tennis partner. Whiter-than-white pleated skirts and frilly knickers are de rigeur. You rarely get a chance to be such a cliché.

Resist the lure of Lycra. It is far cooler to wear baggy old sweats in the gym than a brand-new shiny leotard and thong ensemble. If you are tempted to buy such an ensemble, chances are you are a gym novice. If you wear spanking new, fully branded Lycra leggings and thong-leotard to your first Step class, everyone will know you are a novice. These garments are intended for gym-pros with perfect bodies. No one likes to look like a sausage that is about to burst.

Never wear make-up in the gym. Rivulets of sweat are at least natural, if not exactly attractive. Streaks of foundation and mascara will get you pitying looks. If you do wear make-up to the gym, be sure not to actually raise a sweat when you work out.

Don't join a chi-chi gym where the women are all pencil thin despite seemingly hanging out at the juice bar all day.

Only gay men pick up in the gym.

Forget the gym and go swimming instead. Once you're in no one can tell what size you are. Even the roundest of physiques moves gracefully under water.

Second Skin

The designer Azzedine Alaia, also known as the 'King of Cling' for his range of skin-tight clothing, may well have demanded an impeccable physique for his dresses, but you'll be relieved to hear that being stylish doesn't mean being skinny. It may be true that you can never be too rich, but you certainly can be too thin. We would have been better off lis-

'The base of all beauty is the body.'

— Azzedine Alaia

tening to one of Wallis Simpson's less-quoted aphorisms on style: 'I am not a beautiful woman. The only thing to do is dress better than all the others.'

Instead of looking for clothes you fit into, find clothes that fit you. No one looks good in clothes that don't fit. No matter how expensive or well made. Even a size ten catwalk model squeezed into a size eight sample dress will bulge like a Gladstone bag over the back.

Too-tight t-shirts make your bust look like two pigs wrestling under a blanket.

The psychology of clothes sizing is a minefield. A woman can be a size ten in one shop, but a size fourteen in another. So why do we shoe-horn ourselves into a twelve when we know the fourteen fits so much better? Buy clothes that fit. You can always cut out the label. It is only a label.

47% of the population is a size sixteen or over.

Things a Woman Should Know About Style

Shop in Gap. You'll immediately be wearing clothes two sizes smaller. Until you go to America and everyone else is too. You see, it's all relative. If you are a UK size twelve, for example, in the US you are usually a ten, but try on an eight. (Gap say an eight, but in general subtract just two for your American size). In France you are a forty, but in Italy you are a forty-two. What does a number mean?

If you are in between sizes buy the size up, not the size down. Resist the temptation to grow into it.

Designer clothes are often cut bigger than on the high street (their profit margins allow for extra fabric among other

'A lady, however poor, should wear fine linen —
even if she can only have one new dress a year.'

— Elinor Glyn

things.) This is particularly true of brands aimed at an older market.

No one is a normal size in Top Shop unless you are under fifteen and have a thigh the same width as your knee.

Don't shop in Top Shop if you are over thirty. No matter how tempting a twenty pound look-a-like Prada top is. Ignore people who tell you they can't tell the difference between a fifteen and a fifty pound one. You can. It's not a matter of design, but economics: it's just not viable to put as much fabric or as much manufacturing expertise into a garment that costs a third of the price.

When investing in clothes you intend to have for a long time, remember the following:

- Buy classic styles, not this season's latest power shoulder-pad jacket.

Things a Woman Should Know About Style

- Buy luxury: cashmere twinsets, silk underwear and fine leather shoes.

- Buy one good piece of clothing instead of five badly made ones.

- Please, please buy the right size. Shop for as long as it takes to find clothes that really fit you and have them altered if they don't.

- Never, ever buy clothes you intend to slim into or – oh the possibility of it – gain weight to fill.

- It cannot be emphasised enough – BUY THE RIGHT SIZE!

- Buy simple classic lines that flatter your figure. Subtlety is all if you want your clothes to have style and longevity.

- Have your clothes altered, preferably by a good tailor employed by the store you are buying from. If you are paying a lot of money this is the least you can expect. Even if you are not paying a lot this service should always be available.

'The greatest beauty in female dress is that which is most simple and at the same time gracefully adapted to exhibit the natural beauty of the female form.'

— George Pope Morris

- Use a dressmaker. Find clothes you like and have them tailored to fit you. Better still, find the perfect fit and then have it copied.

- Having clothes made is good for your self-esteem. No numbers, no sales assistants and no communal changing rooms.

Minimalism: Alive and Well

The capsule wardrobe sounds like an urban myth and a boring one at that. It's not. The concept of pared-down basics, sensible separates that all co-ordinate and an absence of embarrassing sale bargains seems unlikely to fit in any world outside that of a minimalist designer boutique. Unlikely yes, impossible no. Re-jigging your clothes to create a personalised capsule wardrobe to fit in with your own style will result in a

'The more you know, the less you need.'

— Australian Aboriginal saying

better wardrobe than an afternoon with your credit card in Joseph, and it's a hell of a lot cheaper.

Still not convinced? It's simple. Pare down your clothes into basics that all co-ordinate with each other and a) you will look better, but b) you will get at least an extra half hour in bed in the morning as any top you grab will go with any bottom.

A cleverly put-together basic wardrobe is the cornerstone of classic style. Build it around a base colour (black is the obvious one, but dark brown or navy work similarly well) and add colours that tone one by one. For example, white, camel, pale blue, etc. Similarly with styles: suits, bootleg trousers, shirts and neat sweaters – or pencil-skirts, twinsets and dresses. Whatever works for you. Don't panic, you can add in your pink frou-frou mules later.

Once you've chucked out clothes that don't fit, clothes you don't like and clothes that belong in the '80s (no sentimentality here) your wardrobe will be pretty basic anyway, and most of it will be black.

The perfect white t-shirt is essential and equally chic worn with jeans or under suits. It is elusive so persevere: look for opacity, stretch and washability. This is one garment that must always be pristine. If you find the perfect fit, buy one, wash it, check it doesn't shrink or bobble then go back and buy ten. You will regret it if you don't and the

Classic style is about clever tailoring, wearing clothes that fit, and the well-thought-out (in advance) use of colour and pattern.

Style also means life-style. There is no point wearing tight, chic dresses, high-heels, a headscarf and dark glasses if you spend the day rushing around from meeting to meeting (unless you are important enough to afford taxis for every 500-yard journey) or playing with your kids. So wear a smart, comfortable shift dress or black stretch trousers, a white shirt and good quality flats to the office, dark jeans and a simple, neat sweater for weekends.

Looking Good
is in Your Jeans

A bad pair of jeans is the least flattering item of clothing in the world. A good pair is the most. Men should never iron jeans, women always should, but not, as some fashions have deemed, with a crease down the front. We're talking a once-over, not a starch effect.

'Fashion' jeans should be avoided at all cost. Why anyone wants to pay hundreds for torn jeans with paint splattered on them is a mystery. I suppose DIY-ing a pair at home with a pot of emulsion is too uncool. Much more fun though. Sequin-adorned, fabric trimmed, patchworked and held together by

Things a Woman Should Know About Style

'I don't know what she does with all the clothes she buys. I only ever see her in blue jeans.'

— Aristotle Onassis on his wife, Jackie

safety pins: these are all examples of fashion's corruption of jeans. No pair of jeans has been safe since Liberty's decided to trim jeans and jackets with their trademark floral prints. An unlikely sartorial marriage if ever there was one.

Jeans can be stylish. Dark blue jeans are the classic choice, but a pair of lovingly faded jeans is beyond reproach. It is as sentimentally important as the comforter blanket you took everywhere as a child.

There is nothing more guaranteed to make you feel good than putting on your favourite pair of jeans.

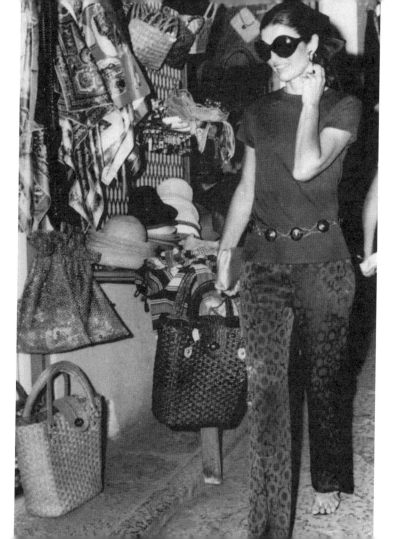

Things a Woman Should Know About Style

'Old clothes are old friends.'

— Coco Chanel

It takes years to wear jeans to just the way you like them. A sure-fire tip for good fading is to wear daily and never wash them. More of a boy's tip, I think. If you find yourself unable to fit into the jeans that were feel-good favourites for so many

Denim was invented in the nineteenth century as an industrial-strength labourers' cloth. Levi-Strauss aimed his first batch of rough, heavy cotton trousers at men who needed resistant clothes to withstand hard work. Jeans were simply a utilitarian garment until the 1950s, when they were popularised by film stars like James Dean and Marilyn Monroe. Having left behind its proletarian origins, denim is unique in being the one fabric that completely transcends gender, class or race.

years, convince yourself that it is they that have shrunk and not you who have grown and kiss them a fond goodbye. Never buy the same brand in a larger size.

Jeans and trainers are not stylish. Jeans and flat loafers are classic. Jeans and high-heels are either very tarty or very 'now' depending on whether you are at an Essex nightclub or an A-list celebrity party. Sometimes it's hard to tell the difference.

Why wear jeans to a party when there are so many fabulous clothes around?

From the Inside Out

Like beauty, being well dressed is all in the eye of the behol-der, but there are certain things you can wear that increase your chances of objectively looking good.

The way clothes make you feel cannot be underestimated when it comes to looking good. The basic trick to pulling off classic

'Understatement has a chic denied to over-empha-sis.'

— Arthur Bauman

'No woman can make herself chic if she is not chic herself.'

— Balenciaga

style is being comfortable in what you are wearing, being yourself and not trying too hard. Or at least looking like you are not trying too hard.

Start with what makes you feel good. Or confident. Or powerful. Or sexy. Or in control. Or all of the above.

Don't be afraid of a uniform. If it works it works. That doesn't mean it can't be stylish. All icons of style have formulas, carefully honed over years. Don't expect to find your formula until you are at least thirty years of age. From then on it'll just get better as you push the boundaries and start to gain more confidence in what you wear. You need to grow into yourself before your clothes will fit perfectly. Sticking to the formula means you don't make mistakes. If you always wear black, so be it. Once you've found a formula that works you can mould it by adding in colours, shapes and so on.

Style should look effortless and fit you. Not everyone suits the same clothes. Think how many times you've seen some to-die-for outfit in a shop but known you could never pull it off? Yet it has your best friend's name written all over it.

Coco Chanel knew that clothes had to fit your lifestyle, and in order to be stylish it is essential you wear the right clothes for your life. If you are reading this book, classic style is what appeals to you, but what kind of classic style? Coco Chanel – smart suits and pearls or Coco Chanel – men's trousers and

'Fashion is not something that only exists in clothes... .it has something to do with ideas, with the way we live, with what happens around us.'

— Coco Chanel

'It is [every woman's] right to ignore the dictates of fashion and dress in a manner that is becoming to her own character and personality.'

— Lillie Langtry

Breton tops? Grace Kelly in pencil skirts and twinsets or Katherine Hepburn in men's-style clothing?

Face the fact that style schizophrenia is not only acceptable, it is inevitable. No one lives the same life or needs the same kind of clothes all the time, even if it is as simple as Madame Chanel's different styles of dress for city and country. Think about what you want. Your style of clothing should be as comfortable as your own skin.

If you're not comfortable in your own skin, you'll never be comfortable in any clothes.

It's a Man's World

If the benchmark of patrician elegance – the 1950s stylised ideal of tailored skirt, twinset and pearls and heels – feels too old-fashioned, find a different ideal. Or create your own. Women are lucky enough today to be able to wear pretty much what they want. Take trousers for example. Imagine a world where you were banned from restaurants, hotels and night-clubs because you were wearing trousers. Or asked to remove the bottom half of your trouser suit, so it seemed you were wearing a micro-mini rather than the forbidden attire of men.

In the 1950s Katharine Hepburn was repeatedly asked to wear a dress rather than trousers when visiting her beau, Spencer Tracy, at Claridges. It was not deemed appropriate for a woman to be seen in a smart hotel in such attire. Outraged, she chose to use the staff entrance to the hotel rather than give up her adored trademark trousers.

As late as 1966, when Yves Saint Laurent designed a female version of his famous tuxedo, wealthy socialites were barred from restaurants and hotels if they were wearing the trouser suit. Instead, they were asked to remove their trousers, and leave their jackets on, so it seemed as if they were wearing a miniskirt. The shortest skirt was preferable to a woman in trousers.

If there is one garment that revolutionised the way women dressed in the twentieth century it has to be trousers. For many women, trousers are more comfortable, more practical and more flattering than skirts. Trousers have been making a modern style statement ever since Chanel wore them in the 1920s and '30s. It is a look that endures to this day.

Wide-legged, fitted at the waist and hips, '30s-style 'sailor pants' are flattering to all figures. If you have wide hips, chunky legs or are just rounded all over, this style will balance your shape. Wear them long enough to cover your shoe.

There is nothing worse than a pair of trousers that are the wrong length. Trousers should fall well onto your shoe – to mid-heel if you are wearing high heels – and should not ride up past your socks when you sit down. This looks bad enough on men, even worse when it reveals a pair of laddered pop-socks on a woman. Properly tailored trousers should be cut slightly higher at the front than at the back. Don't attempt this at home.

When we talk about trousers as 'fitted', we don't mean skin-tight. The aim is to skim lumps and bumps and achieve a smooth and flattering line. It is not to make yourself look like

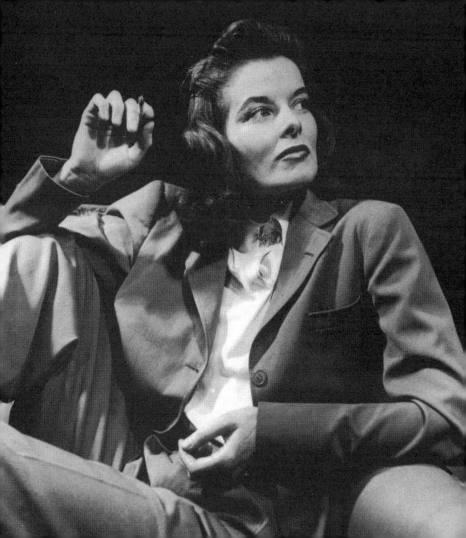

an over-stuffed sofa. Taking out pockets will remove bulk and sewing them up gives trousers a clean line. The same applies to jacket pockets. They are sewn up for a reason. If you un-pick them the fabric begins to sag, and if – crime above all other – you fill your pockets with keys and coins or stuff your hands in, your smart tailored jacket will soon come to resemble a baggy old cardigan.

For real period glamour, wear wide trousers with turn-ups and brogues. Wear tops short with this style of trouser, and shirts tucked in, with a smart belt over them. The waist of your trouser should be high if you are accentuating it – don't bother belting at the hips, you're just doing your figure a disservice.

It is a myth that wearing things tucked in makes you look bigger. In fact the opposite is true – a belt gives you a defined waist and, whatever your size, this is a good thing. A shirt hanging out over wide trousers makes you completely shapeless. Voluptuous hourglass types will particularly benefit from this advice, and look stunning in a pair of wide tailored trousers, a crisp white shirt tightly belted in. If you've got it, flaunt it.

Shirts should fit perfectly! No pulling across the bust, no sleeves too long or too short. Have one tailor-made in the City – even if you don't work there. It is cheaper than you think.

High-waisted trousers make your legs look longer. Add a pair of heels and they'll go on forever.

A shirt is best left hanging out over tight trousers. Choose a slightly fitted, three-quarter length cotton that is long enough to hide a multitude of sins. Cropped capri pants are the epitome of elegance in summer. Think Audrey Hepburn playing 'Moon River' on her balcony in *Breakfast at Tiffany's* wearing capri pants, a shirt and a headscarf more suitable for doing the cleaning in. Improbably yet ineffably chic.

Man-made fibres have been used to make fabric for more than a century. Rayon was invented in the late nineteenth century and began to be commercially produced in America in 1910. Acetate was commercially produced by the 1920s and nylon was hailed as a miracle fabric in 1930. Polyester, acrylic and spandex became well known by the 1960s. Other than rayon and acetate, man-made fibres are unabsorbent.

Spandex is the generic name for all polyurethane fibres. It can stretch to five or more times its own size and immediately contract back to its original shape.

Spandex is a miracle fibre. An average 5–10% spandex in your cotton keeps your clothes in shape and your body under control. In some combinations spandex doesn't machine wash, so check the label or you could get that impossible-to-iron-out wrinkle effect. And if you ever spy little threads poking out of the backside of your trousers throw them out. The spandex has begun to break, the fabric to sag, and from behind you now look like you are wearing a nappy.

Cigarette pants – don't call them drainpipes unless you want to be identified with the 1980s – are the tightest trouser of all. Don't wear them if your legs are too fat – or too thin. A perfect figure is essential.

Boot-leg trousers are a contemporary style that serves the same purpose as the wide-leg. They balance wide hips and flatter big legs. And if you are skinny they will stop you looking like you are held up by a pair of cocktail sticks. Boot-leg means they are designed to go over boots, so don't get a pair that stops at your ankles. A flare of fabric half-way down your calf is not chic. People will think your trousers have shrunk.

Black cotton/spandex boot-leg trousers are a mainstay of the modern woman's wardrobe, so make sure you get a good pair. The fabric should be thick enough so it doesn't bag at the knees (the joy of spandex is that it should spring back into shape when you stand up).

Material Girl

Man-made fibres have their place but natural fabrics are on the whole, better, and more comfortable, to wear. Sweat stains are not a good look.

Natural fibres – linen, cotton, silk and wool – have a distinguished history that is reflected in the clothes made from them. This is, needless to say, in turn reflected in their price.

Wool is said to absorb the smell of sweat, making it the ultimate fabric for bodies prone to perspiration.

Buy expensive clothes made from high-quality fabric but fewer of them. They will last you a lifetime if you choose well. This is, of course, utterly pointless if you come home from a drunken party, having spilt wine down your dress, pull it off without bothering to undo the buttons, thus stretching it, then drop it into the washing basket when you suspect it is dry-clean only. Similarly, screwing up your cashmere cardigan into a ball and pushing it to the back of a moth-infested cupboard till the next time you need to go out in a slip of a dress. Sound familiar?

Take care of your clothes or forget looking good. It is impossible to look stylish in faded, shrunken clothes.

Wash 'n Go

Cotton is in principle machine washable and dry-cleanable. Woven cotton shrinks slightly, knitted cotton shrinks more dramatically. White cotton tends to yellow with age or long-term exposure to sunlight. Short-term exposure to sunlight bleaches white cotton; getting it right is a fine art. Coloured cotton is bleached easily by sunlight and strong detergents. Unfortunately often by dry-cleaners too. Iron hot.

Linen can sustain high temperatures and its fibres are stronger wet than dry. If not pre-shrunk it will shrink significantly when washed, particularly if loose-woven. Good quality linen is expensive so don't take any risks. Have it dry-cleaned or professionally laundered. Don't tumble dry linen – it will probably shrink and if not you will never get the creases out. Iron very hot.

Wool is more delicate to care for. Hand-wash briefly in cool water with a mild detergent. Never wring when wet – the fibres are very weak – instead, roll in a towel and squeeze gently. Wool completely loses its shape when wet. Reshape from memory or, as some guides to household management suggest, draw an outline before washing it! Dry flat on a towel away from direct heat or sunlight. Iron cool.

Any wool that is machine washable has been pre-treated with chemicals to make it that way. To be safe, have wool dry-cleaned. Accidentally machine-washed wool that has gone solid and shrunk to half its size can sometimes be resurrected by soaking in cold water and gently pulling back into shape.

Cashmere: there is great debate as to whether to dry-clean or hand-wash cashmere. The more delicate the treatment the better. Hand-washing in shampoo is recommended by aficionados.

A cavalier attitude to cleaning clothes is tantamount to adopting a 'wear it once, throw it away' wardrobe philosophy. Read the label and take heed. Plenty of manufacturers do put 'dry-clean only' on most clothes as a disclaimer, but are you willing to take the risk? Check your whole garment is machine washable before chucking it in the machine. Trims and linings may not be.

If you follow the washing instructions on the label and something shrinks, pulls or fades badly take it back to the store for a replacement or your money back. Always keep receipts for expensive clothes. You shouldn't need them but in general the more exclusive and expensive the garment the snottier and less helpful the sales assistants become when you try to return it. A miraculous transformation from the day you were charmed in to buying it.

If you dry-clean an item and it comes back the worse for wear, resign yourself to an on-going battle between cleaner and store as to who is to blame. It is very unlikely anyone will take responsibility. Avoid the above scenario: find yourself a good dry-cleaner.

Going Undercover

Finding clothes that fit is first and foremost when it comes to having style, and good foundation garments are most important of all. Buy a corset – your grandmother would be proud of you.

Today there is no excuse for wearing a bra that doesn't fit, when you can buy a good bra relatively cheaply. Get measured professionally; it is almost impossible to get it right yourself and department stores will do it for free.

If facing the no-nonsense fitters at the likes of Rigby and Peller (think Hattie Jacques in *Carry On* films) is just too much, you

A 1920s flapper had strict instructions as to what to wear under her skimpy flapper dress: 'bust flattener brassiere and corset with adjustable straps, back-stitched front panel, elasticised side and back panel, side fastenings with hooks and bars and four adjustable garters, along with a lace-trimmed crepe-de-Chine slip.' (From a product description of 1926 in *A Century of the Designer* by Charlotte Seeling [Konemann].)

can roughly measure yourself as follows: Measure around your back beneath the bust. This is your back size, for example, 34 inches. Now measure around the fullest part of the bust. The difference between them should give you a rough idea of your cup-size. A five-inch difference is roughly a C-cup. Add or subtract as necessary.

All bras fit differently. There is only one way to find the right bra. Try it on. Here's how: do it up at the back on the first hook. The bra will loosen with wear, which is the only time you will go down to the second or third set of hooks. If you find the innermost hook fits better when it's new, go down a whole back size – from 36 to 34, for example. (If you go down from a 36C, you will need a 34D, the cup being proportionate to the back. Similarly if you go up a cup size, from 34C to D, you will automatically get more room around the back).

Now, making sure no one is watching, lean forward, lift up the breast and drop it into the cup. Unglamorous, but essential. Next – and this is where an experienced fitter comes in handy, tighten the straps. A fitter will wrench the strap down your back in the style of a Victorian lady's maid tightening a corset, forcing you to throw your shoulders back with military precision. A tug and a lift later and the bra should be on. Any gaps at the sides of the cup and it is too big; any bulges, it is too small.

A new bra will feel tight across the back. Tighter than you are used to perhaps, but remember that new bras are like new shoes, they always leave marks the first time you wear them. A few wears and a hand-wash will soon loosen it up.

Always hand-wash underwired bras. Unless you want to pay for a new washing machine drum.

For most of us a gentle bulge beneath the bra is one of the inevitabilities of not being a model. Too much of a bulge, particularly over the top and sides of the cup, brings to mind rolls of uncooked dough and unsavoury similes involving lard. This is one time that you don't want your cup to spilleth over.

How to make a bra look good: stand up straight. Shoulders back, breasts out.

Buy bras in black, white and nude. Accept the fact that nude underwear is not sexy. Console yourself that it will disappear when you wear white or sheer clothing. It is obvious that black underwear will shine through white

'Brevity is the soul of lingerie.'

— Dorothy Parker

cloth, but few people realise that white shows through just as clearly.

The faint shadow of a lacy white bra under a crisp white shirt has a certain European sexiness about it. This is the only time a visible white bra looks stylish. Black bras should only ever be seen under sheer black chiffon evening shirts, and then only if you have a perfect figure. A bulging tummy between bra and belt is not a pleasant sight.

The fashion for underwear as outerwear should be avoided at all costs.

· 77 ·

Don't think you look hip and happening if you have a coloured bra-strap on show under your camisole top or peeking out of an off-the-shoulder blouse. Only teenagers can get away with this kind of thing.

Red underwear may say things about you that you don't want other people to hear. According to certain underwear boutiques, men find red lace sexy. Women, on the other hand, find it tarty. Electric blue, lime green, neon pink or anything in nylon or polyester: don't go there unless you are having a '70s-throw-back moment.

Crotchless or nipple-less underwear is taking things too far. Forget the decency question, just imagine the draughts. What would your mother say? ('Always wear clean knickers, dear, you never know when you might get run over.')

Lace underwear is beautiful but scratchy, silk underwear is sexy but lacks support, cotton underwear is chaste (apparently) and seamless underwear is boring but essential.

Bust-enhancing bras have their place, but don't wear them beneath clothing that is not completely opaque or everyone will see the pads. Very embarrassing. (This is also worth remembering if you are breastfeeding and using breast-pads!) Never, ever stick tissue-paper in your bra. It is an advertising gimmick that loo-paper is suitable for this purpose. Have you ever seen a pair of square boobs?

If going without, do as the stars do: hoist 'em and stick 'em with toupe tape. Don't try this if you are over a B-cup. Toupe tape is really just double-sided Sellotape.

G-Strings or Big Pants?

G-strings look great under clothes but awful in the flesh. Dental floss, wedgie or cheese-wire are apt descriptions of its comfort rating. It is depressing to pay more for five square inches of Lycra than you do for ten, nevertheless the VPL or Visible Panty Line is the well-dressed woman's nemesis. Grin and wear it.

Big pants have a certain Berlin-stripper appeal, just make sure they are big enough. There is nothing worse than bottoms bulging over knicker elastic.

Things a Woman Should Know About Style

Wear G-strings under trousers, big pants under flowing skirts and nothing under skin-tight dresses. Invest in tights with built in gusset.

Avoid wearing no underwear under a short dress unless you can guarantee sitting still in one place, legs demurely crossed. Above all never walk up a staircase if you have no underwear on.

'If skirts get any shorter,'
Said the flapper with a sob
'There'll be two more cheeks to powder
And one more place to "bob". - James Laver
(Quoted in the *Pimlico Companion to Fashion*)

Alternatively think big: tummy-sucking waist-cinching panties, thigh-slimming, bottom-lifting tights and anything with the word 'control' in its description are the guardians of the pear-shaped woman's vanity. Don't be alarmed if you are striped red and white and half your usual size when you take these things off. It's a bit like coming up from a deep-sea dive: you have to re-pressurise gradually.

Tights should be gusset-less for slinky dresses, toe-less for sandals and virtually sheer for the perfect finish over naked legs. Ultra-sheer black for black dresses, nude for any other colour. Never buy anything that describes itself as American Tan.

Resign yourself to the fact that 7-denier tights will only last an evening, if you're lucky. Always carry a spare pair in your bag. Expensive 7-denier tights don't last longer than cheap ones they just look better for the few hours before you ladder them. Beware of ragged nails, rings, rough skin, car upholstery and antique chairs when trying to keep your tights ladder-free.

Stockings make you feel sexy, men go wild for them (apparently) and they are more hygienic. Suspender belts, on the other hand, are fiddly and lumpy. Hold-ups may be the answer, even if they are reminiscent of support-stockings. You also run the risk of embarrassing pings of elastic. Very *Bridget Jones*.

In Victorian England upper-class women were expected to call on as many as four or five acquaintances for afternoon tea... and then go on to dinner, wearing corsets that squashed internal organs into half their required space. Women mastered the art of subtly picking at their food, as this was both considered ladylike as well as the only way to avoid a disten-ded stomach, unthinkable in such restrictive clothing.

Before a really big party a body-wrap that promises to 'take off inches' actually will take you down a dress size or so. It won't last – you will have swelled back up to your usual size by the following morning. A DIY cling-film wrap at home will not, unfortunately, have the same effect. You'll just sweat a lot and get very sticky.

Tight frocks and social events that involve eating are mutually exclusive. Unfortunately, starving yourself for a day is more likely to leave you bloated than stick-thin. Plus you'll have bad breath. Eat moderately before you go.

Get your priorities straight: good food before fashion every time.

Alternatively, wear a stylish Eastern-inspired voluminous tunic and trouser ensemble. (This also works a treat when pregnant.)

Ladies Lounge

Up until the 1950s, the words 'why don't you slip into something more comfortable?' didn't just sound like a bad line from *Dallas*. Wafting around the house in a beautiful silk gown was perfectly acceptable and desperately stylish.

There formally existed a kind of wonderfully elegant structured silk pyjama for evening or beach wear. Bring it on! All in favour of re-introducing the trend start building your wardrobe of dressing gowns immediately. Personal favourites include deep pink satin, marl grey cashmere and a vintage gold 1950s Chinese number complete with buttons and shoulder pads. Now that's a housecoat. Forget those nylon eyesores so popular in the '60s.

Pyjamas and nightwear in general have a big role to play in the style icon's wardrobe. Minimalists and harassed mothers should buy white and beige linen pyjamas: you may be crumpled but at least you can claim to be wearing the latest in Eastern chic.

Nightwear is a place to live out your style-icon fantasies. Silk negligees and matching robes have a Jean Harlow-esque glamour. Put on your bleached blond wig and curl up on the sofa watching old movies and eating Charbonel and Walker violet and rose creams.

In movie-land where nothing ever creases, sirens sleep in silk or satin nighties. In the real world you will resemble a wrung-out dishrag in the morning, and I always find myself battling to turn over in the night, hindered by moist fabric stuck firmly to the underside of my body, refusing to budge.

Better still, sleep naked. Bit cold in winter, though.

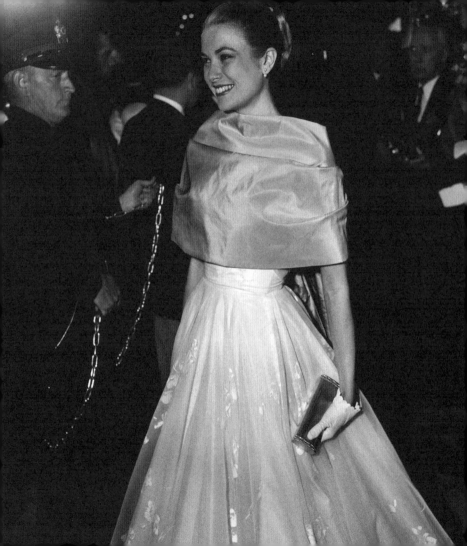

You Shall
Go to the Ball!

A big party, a hot date, the beginning of summer or the end of a hard week at work are all excellent excuses for dressing up. These are the times that you really need to know how to pull off screen-diva glamour. Good underwear may be the foundation of a fantastic outfit, but don't spoil it with what you put over the top. Once in a while give in to the little girl inside every sober career woman who can't resist a floor-length silver sequin-encrusted evening gown. On all other occasions wear black.

'Getting dressed and going out is fun only because we don't do it often – it's good to feel glamorous once in a while.'

— Adolfo, fashion designer

The capsule evening wardrobe: Black cocktail dresses (in fact as many little black dresses as you can collect) for all occasions; cream or subtly coloured silk blouses, beaded tops and/or more risqué items such as backless or halter-neck tops depending on your age and shape – all to be worn with smart, wool crêpe black trousers for dinners and cocktail parties; plenty of high-heeled shoes; dresses: light and shimmery for summer; heavy and shiny for formal; bright, bold and flattering of figure for feeling fantastic anytime.

As long as an outfit fits your body, flatters your complexion and you have the personality to carry it off you can get away with almost anything. Confidence is all. If you are in doubt, a black dress will usually make you feel confident and almost always look stylish, even if it didn't cost a lot of money.

A good dress will make you feel sexy, confident and fabulous about your body.

Beware of the effect on drunken men a sexy dress can have. Be pleased with any effect a dress has on a sober man.

There is a fine line to be drawn between over-cautious and over-flamboyant dressing. Err too much on the side of little black dress and you will fade into the anonymous masses of other women in little black dresses. Yet it is a brave woman who wears red to a party of sniffy social X-rays dressed in black.

'A dress has no meaning unless it makes a man want to take it off.'

— Francois Sagan

Things a Woman Should Know About Style

Always check out dress codes before you go:

Smart/Casual: An all-purpose, annoyingly ambiguous dress code that has become the norm for drinks or dinner parties. People tend to concentrate on either the smart bit or the casual bit, but a suit is too smart and jeans and trainers are too casual. Chanel-style smart pleated trousers and a cashmere sweater are the height of smart/casual chic.

Cocktail: Strappy dress or trouser suit and heels depending on your mood.

Lounge Suits: A terrible, 1970s-sounding dress code that people offer as an alternative to black tie on invitations if they are worried you don't have a tuxedo. Make your man wear his best suit, but with a t-shirt not a shirt and tie. Still cocktail garb for girls.

Black Tie: Whoever said feminism was alive and well wasn't referring to fashion. Men get away with wearing the same tuxedo for twenty years but women are criticised if they wear the same dress twice. If you are only buying one formal dress, buy a timeless black, then if you get the opportunity splash out on fabulous coloured frocks for special occasions.

Alternatively, women's tuxedos *à la* Marlene Dietrich have come back in vogue of late. Stylish, but you run the risk of being mistaken for a man. Only really works at very trendy parties so don't try it at your parents golden wedding anniversary.

White Tie: The most formal of dress codes, latterly known as 'white tie and tiaras', is virtually obsolete outside the ranks of royalty, diplomats and Elton John's annual soirées. Officially it means a stiff starched white collar, white bow-tie and tails for

'Suitability is half the secret of being well-dressed.'

— Mainbocher

men, long ballgowns and jewels for women, but unless you are invited to a state occasion it is unlikely anyone is going to be checking.

Never pass up an opportunity to wear a tiara.

Fancy Dress: Guaranteed to make your heart plummet when you read the invitation, but it's a Catch 22. If you don't try you look like a killjoy, if you do, you look plain stupid. If in doubt, hire a professional costume. Expensive, but worth it.

If everyone else is hiring professional costumes, wear the first thing you find in the dressing-up box and doctor it accordingly. Make sure everyone knows you have genuinely entered into the spirit of things rather than paid for the easy option.

Quickly get your own back: have a '70s party.

You Shall Go to the Ball!

Be kind, have a '20s party. Terribly glamorous in a Gatsby-ish kind of way. Not so good if you are blessed with big bosoms.

A fancy dress party is one of the few times that even the little black dress won't work.

The Little Black Dress

The little black dress is truly a style essential, but when you walk into a room full of other little black dresses – and you will, plenty of times – your little black dress needs to stand out.

If you think a little black dress is just a little black dress, think again. There are as many permutations of black dresses as there are moods you might want to wear one for.

For classic day-wear, lunching or garden parties wear the fitted black shift dress. Slashed neckline, skimming, not clinging to the contours of the body, dropping to just below the knee.

The Little Black Dress

Think Audrey Hepburn wearing Givenchy in *Breakfast at Tiffany's*. A wide-brimmed hat, with a cream satin trim and a pair of high-heeled slingbacks complete the illusion that you are a film star.

For slinky evening-wear, make-or-break dates, or landmark birthday parties (how better to feel fabulous at forty?) wear the strappy, ruched black dress. Heart-shaped bodice, closely fitted but made from clever, rippled fabric that conceals lumps and bumps, it ends just on the knee to reveal finely shaped calves clad in impossibly sheer black tights. Think Marilyn Monroe

'You can wear black at any time, you can wear it at any age, you may wear it on almost any occasion. A "little black frock" is essential to a woman's wardrobe. I could write a book about black.'

— Christian Dior

or Jessica Rabbit. Accessorise with a pair of vertiginous black satin Manolos with a discreet and feminine little bow on them. This is the outfit to get – or keep – your man in.

Other useful little black dresses include the black shift dress for the office; the black linen shirt dress for summer; the wrap-around silk jersey for informal events you still want to look smart at; the stretchy, forgiving black dress for days you feel fat, but need to look slim.

That black holds centre stage in timeless style can be attributed to Chanel, who in 1919 gave black its fashion credentials. She on claimed it all stemmed from a charity ball where she perceived the colours the women were wearing as 'too awful, they make the women ugly. I think they ought to be dressed in black.'

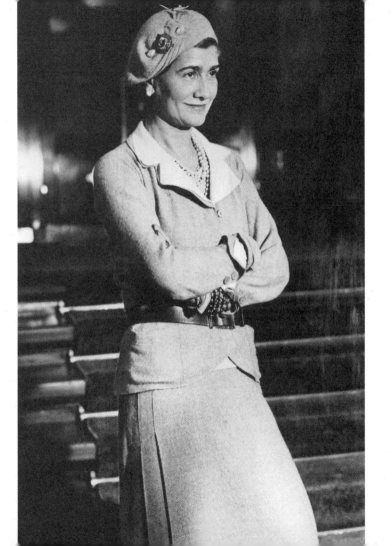

Black in Style

Black is every woman's safety net.

Black makes you look taller and thinner.

Black is timelessly chic.

'Women who wear black lead colourful lives.'

— Neiman Marcus advertisement

Black will take you anywhere. Except to a wedding. Unless you are Liza Minnelli, who at her wedding to David Guest had a dozen bridesmaids wearing black. Is this a good omen, we ask?

The best way to make black less obviously black is to mix it with white.

Never wear a black hat to a wedding. Even if everyone else is. Everyone else may be. Everyone else is wrong.

The only formal occasion to which you should wear black is a funeral.

Make the most of weddings, days at the races and garden parties; an excuse to wear colour at last.

There is never a 'new black'. Black is the only black. But there are some places where other colours might as well be black they are so ubiquitous. Navy blue: black for the upper middle classes. Dark brown: black for country aristocrats.

> In 1910, when the country was in mourning for Edward VII, the Ascot race meeting of that year became legendary, known as 'Black Ascot'. Women had the latest styles made up in black and mourning became a fashion statement.

Red: black for fashion editors when they just can't bear black any longer.

Christian Lacroix was right when he said there are many different shades of black. This is very annoying, particularly when you try to match a black shirt to a black skirt or a black t-shirt to black trousers. Black cotton is a different colour to black silk, black wool or black linen. But black cotton is also a different colour to other black cotton. Black cotton and black linen are the two worst culprits for fading to an unappealing sludge grey.

'Black is the beginning of everything… without it the other colours don't exist. There are many different shades of black.'

— Christian Lacroix

If you can afford it have your black clothes dry-cleaned to pr serve the colour. This is not infallible, however. If black clothes have faded, those magic dye powders that you put in the machine work wonders at restoring density of colour.

Washed-out black is unforgiveable. It is a non-colour.

Washed-out black makes your clothes look old, even if they are not.

Any colour that describes itself as 'washed out' should be avoided. It is usually about as flattering as a washed-out

Things a Woman Should Know About Style

'It is tiresome everlastingly to wear black, but nothing is so serviceable, nothing so unrecognisable, nothing looks so well on every occasion.'

— Emily Post, American socialite, 1922

complexion. In fact anything that lays claim to a 'wash' or 'dye' of any sort should be avoided if you are aiming high in the style stakes. For example, stone-wash, marble-wash, tie-dye.

Let's face it, black is anonymous, that's why we love it so much.

In the Pink

The only colours that have as chic yet as camouflaging an effect as black are white and beige. Wear them in summer when black is just too, well, black. Colour, on the other hand, makes you stand out. Colour is a minefield of potential style errors.

What if the colour doesn't suit you? What if it isn't in fashion? What if it clashes with the other colours you are wearing or with your complexion? What if it sends signals you don't want to send?

Things a Woman Should Know About Style

Never listen to a colour therapist. Particularly if they work under the banner of 'Colour Me Beautiful'. Being told your complexion is Spring therefore you should wear pastels is yet another relic of the '80s that we can do without.

Red is one of the strongest – and carefully chosen, most stylish – colours you can wear. It is the colour of danger and aggression, the colour of sexual predators. Never wear red to an interview.

Red is also a colour that proclaims fiery independence. You either love it or you hate it. Really stylish women love it because they know how to wear it. No one will forget you if you wear red.

Make sure you get the right shade of red. Blue skin-tones should wear blue-based reds. Yellow skin tones should go for more orange reds. Red skin-tones should not wear red. Black women are blessed with being able to wear the brightest reds and oranges and yellows too.

'I can't imagine becoming bored with red — it would be like becoming bored with the person you love.'

— Diana Vreeland

If you are prone to blushing never wear a red polo-neck.

Colour should be appropriate to your environment. If you are going to a garden party or a gentrified summer wedding, wear pastels, not heavy colours like black or red.

We are chameleons at heart: there is nothing so threatening as not fitting in. But some of us are peacocks, desperate to show off the colours of our tail feathers.

There are few classic colours: cream, black and navy blue spring to mind. Lately fashion has proposed that fuschia pink become a classic colour. The jury is still out.

At Your Own Risk

Pattern is even riskier than colour. Be cautious.

Stripes: Horizontally they are nautical and classically stylish for summer beach-resort wear. Vertically they are masculine and business-like; pinstripes are only stylish in a very Marlene Dietrich, hard-nosed kind of way. Not for anyone without chiselled bone structure and slicked-back hair.

Herringbone and Houndstooth: Good if small and classic black and white. It takes a lot to pull off a large and bold houndstooth check, but possible if you are old and slightly eccentric, have a title or at least a smart London address and wear string upon string of real pearls.

Never wear brightly coloured plaids or checks, even if Chanel does make them. The women who wear pink plaid suits are the same women who are tempted by two-tone gold and cream ballet slippers. Faces pulled taught by too many face-lifts, small dog in matching plaid coat squirming to get out of Hermes bag.

Plaids: Only in Scotland. Now that Burberry have succumbed to fashion overkill, the once-understated style of a plaid-lined mackintosh has been lost. Put away your Burberry scarf, or Burberry umbrella and never, ever wear a Burberry-check hat.

If you already have a Burberry mac – considered stylish since *Casablanca* – wear it closed and absolutely don't turn the cuffs back. Casually wrap it around yourself and knot the belt if it gives you enough slack. Take solace in the fact that you had one first.

Polka dots: Keep them very small for society events.

Animal prints: Reminiscent of East End madams and the cover of a Jackie Collins novel. Risky, unless of course you are in Italy. When in Rome…

Flowers: If you're going floral do it big and bold, Barbados-style on a brightly coloured caftan, preferably reclining and sipping a cocktail *à la* Princess Margaret. Anything smaller is very domestic.

Wild Pucci prints: In St Tropez, definitely. Always stylish but only if they are genuine. A favourite of Jackie Onassis.

Colour and print is a minefield of potential faux pas. Is it any wonder we always wear black?

Of late, it has become fashionable among the style cognoscenti to substitute the big white dress for the little black dress for a bolder impact. Approach the big white dress with extreme caution. The effect you are aiming for is an Oscar-nominee floor-length gown in luminous white satin. Not a giant snowball. Unless you have the figure of an Oscar-nominated actress stick to the little black dress.

Like a Virgin

The only time a big white dress becomes essential is at a wedding. Your own, never someone else's.

Wedding dresses are horribly, unfairly expensive. Your wedding dress may well be the most expensive dress you ever buy. And you will only wear it once.

To work out the true value of clothes divide the cost of an outfit by the number of times you wear it. For example the most expensive handbag can be justified easily as after all you carry it daily. According to this rule, wedding dresses are very, very bad value. Accept it. Retailers have got you over a barrel. The pictures will be with you for life and it is worth paying any amount of money to look decent on the mantelpiece.

There is something seductive about a wedding outfit that makes budgets go out of the window, for guests as well as brides. At least as a guest you can believe you might wear more than once the horribly expensive dress you buy to make up for the fact your best friend is getting married and you don't even have a boyfriend.

If you are invited to three weddings in a summer, only wear the same dress if it is with three different sets of friends.

The most magnanimous thing a bride can do is resist dressing her bridesmaids in frothy peach confections. Have a heart and choose them a nice dress: they won't upstage you. Remember they are in the pictures too. To be safe, don't have bridesmaids over the age of nine. And don't squeeze plump ones into too-tight dresses. Particularly not pink dresses. They will not thank you when they are older and see themselves immortalised looking like a fat, undercooked sausage.

Things a Woman Should Know About Style

Don't be tempted to think you can dye your wedding dress afterwards. Your wedding shoes, on the other hand, you must definitely dye. Professionally – go back to the store you bought them from for advice.

If you are mercenary, there are agencies that will have your horribly expensive designer gown sold second-hand before you even get back from honeymoon. Slightly distasteful, but let's face it, you're unlikely to see whoever bought it wearing it.

To keep your wedding dress from rotting away Miss Haversham style, have it professionally packed in acid-free tissue paper.

Women shopping for wedding dresses are not rational creatures. They will pay anything, far more than they can afford, to avoid the utter humiliation that is looking bad on your wedding day. If only it were that easy. Take a friend with you. If nothing else you'll have a laugh.

It should be enough to put you off that big wedding dresses are nicknamed meringues. Try one on anyway, just to reassure yourself it looks hideous. Preferably one in nylon so you are not even in the slightest bit tempted. Have a laugh – take a Polaroid. Burn it when you get home.

Shopping for a wedding dress is like shopping for an engagement ring: try on all the ones you will never ever in a million years be able to afford and then have the one you like best copied.

It is a myth that a voluminous wedding dress will disguise a fuller figure or an unannounced pregnancy. You are better off in a flattering, tummy-skimming straight-cut gown. It is claimed that all women lose weight in the run up to their wedding. Don't count on it.

Try on every dress before you decide. It is always the least likely ones that look good.

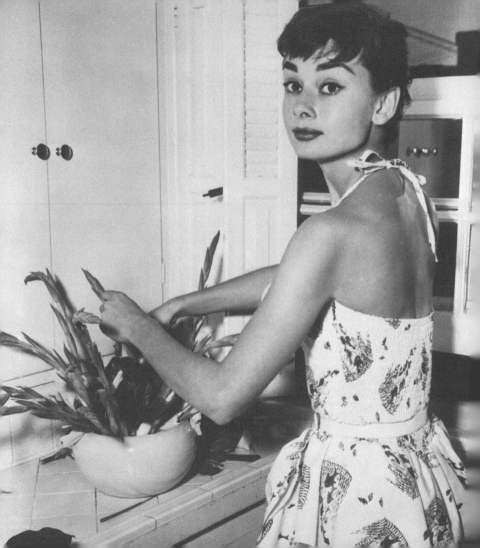

Dressed to Perfection

Good dresses – and this is true of all dresses – tend to look like nothing special on the hanger but fantastic on, and vice versa. A dress that looks stunning on the hanger is unlikely to look so flattering on. This is because real women are not shaped like dress-hangers.

A dress will only look good when it fits properly. If you are paying a lot of money a dressmaker should fit an off-the-peg dress to your exact measurements. And re-fit it if you are not happy.

Things a Woman Should Know About Style

'The dress must not hang on the body but follow its
lines. It must accompany its wearer and when a
woman smiles, her dress should smile with her.'

— Madeleine Vionnet

The perfect dress is the spin-doctor of fashion. It twists and contorts reality into what everyone wants to see.

Dresses are the epitome of style. If you never usually wear one, but want to metamorphose yourself into a lady, try one on. There is no body shape that doesn't benefit from the right dress. Tall and lanky, pick a knee-skimming bias cut. Short and squat: a classic shift with matching jacket.

Never be afraid to take clothes in, let them out, lengthen sleeves or shorten hems. The cornerstone of style is well-fitting clothes. It is a myth that a model figure will fit into any dress.

Turn her around and her back is full of pins. The same is true of actresses. Weeks of costume fittings make that dress look that good.

Once you have the right backdrop, play around with some flourishes. When Patsy Stone (the caricature fashion editor played by Joanna Lumley in the television series *Absolutely Fabulous*) was asked for her top fashion tip she managed, though rigid with fear at her appearance on live television, to splutter the word 'accessories'. It was supposed to be a spoof but she had a point.

'There is no doubt a new dress is a help under all circumstances.'

— Noël Streatfield

You're Never too Fat for Your Handbag

Accessories are to girls what DIY gadgets are to boys. Gratifying for a while but you always want a newer model.

A pair of shoes, a handbag, a scarf or a piece of jewellery can transform you, making you feel like an icon of style. As shoes or bags are, relatively speaking, cheaper than a whole outfit, you might even be able to afford a carbon copy of your real style icon. Chanel sunglasses, Hermes scarves, Manolo Blahnik shoes and Louis Vuitton handbags are all cases in point.

You're Never too Fat for Your Handbag

You never get too fat for your accessories. Although it has been reported by some friends that their feet have swelled two sizes during pregnancy and only gone down one afterwards. Every woman's worst nightmare!

Accessories are the fastest way to buy into designer style, something the designer fashion houses are quick to capitalise on, hence the cult of the handbag. Think everything from the Hermes 'Kelly' Bag to J.P. Tods' 'D' Bag to Fendi's 'baguette'.

Scarves and sunglasses are best for achieving film-star glamour. Think Grace Kelly or Jackie Onassis in a silk Hermes headscarf and a pair of over-sized sunglasses.

Headscarves are tricky. Good if you do look like Grace Kelly, less good if you look like the Queen out shooting in the coun- try. Scarves should look like they were thrown casually around your neck and just happened to fall in a stylish knot. They should not look like you have tried to garrotte yourself on the way over. Isadora Duncan is not a good role model.

Things a Woman Should Know About Style

However you knot your scarf, always wear it with confidence. No one really knows the right way to tie a scarf. Except perhaps the staff in Hermes, who will very kindly show clever ways to make your eighteen-inch square of silk into everything from a choker to a bikini. They also produce a booklet on how to knot – free of charge, which is just as well considering their scarves are pushing two hundred pounds.

Beware of using a scarf as a halter-neck top if you are over eighteen.

Silk scarves are timeless and very classically stylish, but they are ever so slightly stuffy, so wait till you are thirty or have had children before buying one. Pashminas should be timeless, but are still suffering from the fashion overkill that hit a couple of years ago.

A pashmina neatly knotted at the neck says City Trader. A pashmina untidily wound round over a denim jacket says Wannabe Model. A pashmina draped elegantly over the

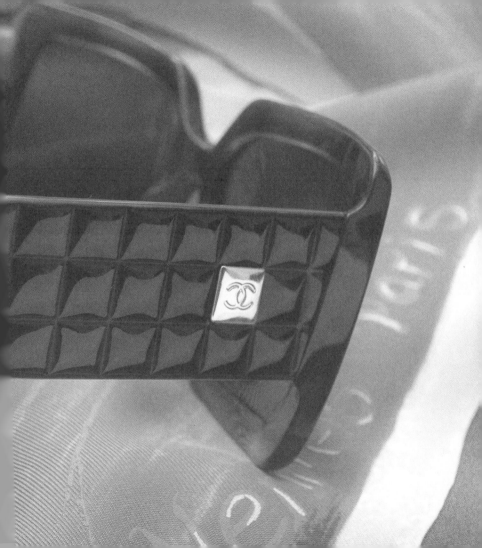

Things a Woman Should Know About Style

shoulders at a Black Tie dinner says Affluent Wife and Mother. A pashmina draped fully over the shoulders in the style of granny's shawl says Cold Fashion Editor, fed up with waiting for another bloody catwalk show to start, three hours late.

Never have your pashmina dry-cleaned, the knots at the end have a tendency to unravel. Wash it – along with the rest of your cashmere – in shampoo instead.

Pashminas are invaluable if you are a new mother and find yourself needing to breastfeed in public.

Sunglasses: don't wear them in the dark or at night. You won't be able to see.

Fashion editors and film stars only wear sunglasses at shows and premieres because they don't want to see. Mostly they are asleep.

Why is it that wearing sunglasses in winter is ridiculed for being desperately try-hard when the sun really is brighter on sunny winter days? A good excuse anyway.

If the Cap Fits

For special occasions the only serious accessory to wear is a hat.

Hats come in all shapes and sizes. It is nonsense to say 'hats don't suit me'. There is a hat to suit every head.

Wide up-swept brims, with scarves trailing behind them in the wind are very classic in an Audrey Hepburn kind of way, but work best if you have an Audrey Hepburn kind of face. Tall, masculine hats are a modern twist on classic style and can be worn with the same structured shift dress as the Audrey hat, this time with a matching long jacket over the top.

Make sure your hat matches your frock. Failing that, a subtle colour difference is more noticeable and more difficult to get away with than a big one. If it is bold you can always claim you did it on purpose. Do so with authority and you will be safe.

Make sure your hat fits. Too small, perched on the crown or too big so you have to keep pushing it out of your eyes are no good. A hat should be comfortable.

'A woman's hat is close to her heart, though she wears it on her head. It is her way of saying to the world, "See this is what I am like – or this is what I would like to be."'

— Lily Dache

Things a Woman Should Know About Style

> *'If you are going to wear a hat at all, be decisive and go the whole hat. In making a courageous choice of millinery, you have nothing to lose but your head.'*

> — *The Bedside Guardian*, 1962

Hats pose a problem for hair, particularly at events like weddings when you will have to take your hat off and be photographed. Long hair is easy: scrape back into a low elegant chignon and your hat sits happily on a smooth scalp. Short hair that fits into the crown is also easy. Mid-length hair is tricky. Try to avoid rogue strands poking out like bits of hay from a haystack or the dreaded bowl imprint when you take off your hat. Best to balance it gently but remember to hold on when gusts of wind come your way.

Be bold: possessing the biggest hat in church is an important achievement.

Dripping with Class

The most enduring accessory of all is jewellery. Jewellery should be acquired over a lifetime of inheritance, extravagance and self-indulgence. Buy carefully or cheaply. Preferably don't buy for yourself at all.

Good rocks are always stylish.

Pearls are the one item of jewellery essential to a style icon's wardrobe. Where would Audrey Hepburn, Grace Kelly or the Queen be without her pearls? Worn under a white shirt for

Things a Woman Should Know About Style

> Natural pearls are the most sought after and valuable and are extremely rare. The demand for these perfect specimens has far out-stripped the supply. Only one percent of pearls are natural and rarely come onto the open market. Instead most common pearls are cultured.

lunch or over a black dress for cocktails, a good set of pearls will make an outfit.

Pearls should be the last thing on and the first thing off. Make-up, lotions and perfume will all discolour pearls, which are prized for their whiteness.

Keep your pearls hanging on the knob of your dresser or the handle of your door. They need moisture in the environment to maintain their lustre and won't take kindly to being boxed away. If you are hanging pearls all over the place, do it high – out of the reach of wandering toddler hands.

Best of all, wear them. Pearls warm to the oils in your skin, gaining lustre and 'dropping' their weight with wear.

Wear them anytime – whoever said pearls and pyjamas wasn't a good look? Lounging around in pearls and silk pyjamas eating chocolates and watching old movies. Now that's style.

Pearls are expensive, around £1,000 for a sixteen-inch neck-lace. A perfect gift from your lover. Forget that – we're modern women: a perfect gift, from (and to) yourself. Costume pearls, however, are perfectly acceptable. Jackie Onassis wore her fake pearls with pride. As long as you look like you can afford real ones, few will tell the difference.

'You can turn an absolute whore in to a lady by just putting pearls around her neck.'

— Donald Brooks

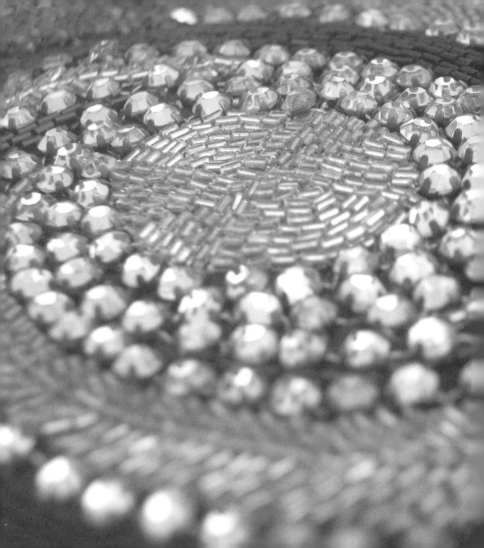

Women have always worn what we now term 'costume jewellery': decorative pieces of jewellery made out of commonplace or semi-precious materials. In the twentieth century the term was coined to refer to pieces designed as a complement to specific outfits. As transitory pieces, costume jewellery is often more flamboyant than valuable jewellery, worn to be flaunted and enjoyed, not hidden away for safe-keeping.

Costume jewellery has just as classic a tradition as valuable jewellery: actresses, society hostesses and royals have collected costume jewellery as avidly as genuine pieces. Diana, Princess of Wales was a big fan.

The best kind of costume jewellery is original. Vintage finds are particularly gratifying. Buying a brooch in Accessorise doesn't quite count. Search your mother's and grandmother's attics: there is bound to be something they have discarded that you can resurrect and flaunt as a family heirloom. An excellent tip for impoverished wannabe style icons.

Things a Woman Should Know About Style

The four main precious stones are diamonds, sapphires, emeralds and rubies. All these stones have long been shrouded in superstition, believed to possess properties far beyond their simple physical beauty.

Sapphires are favoured in the western world because their colouring is so sympathetic to the complexions of northern women. But in the Middle and Far East a sapphire is thought to be either extremely lucky or unlucky. Inconveniently, it is not until you wear it that you know which!

Emeralds are thought to be unlucky because green is associated with bad luck in many cultures. But in ancient Egypt they were used as a healing stone and some believe it has a re-balancing effect on the psyche, even promoting clairvoyancy.

Rubies have always created superstition because they are the colour of blood. In the Far East they are thought to protect the wearer against force and illness. Sometimes referred to as the 'King of Precious Stones', the ruby is associated with fiery temperaments and high energy.

Buy semi-precious stones set with good paste: the untutored eye often can't tell the difference. Besides, paste and costume jewellery is fast becoming valuable in its own right. Pretty semi-precious stones to look for include aquamarine, topaz, coral and amber. Beware of wearing ropes of amber beads: they show a tendency toward hippy eccentricity.

Jewellery is an extremely personal accessory. Whichever style or stone you favour sends a loud and clear message about who you are or who you want to be. Think about it: do you want to be known as a big earring girl or not?

There is something very, very seductive about knowing you have thousands of pounds of jewels about your person. It gives you a tingly feeling quite unlike any other. Make sure they are all insured.

Diamonds really are a girl's best friend.

Especially big ones.

Formed from pure carbon, diamond's complex crystal structure makes it harder than any other stone. Treasured since ancient times, it is only in the last century, with increased mining, that diamonds have become plentiful enough to be worn by commoners as well as royalty. Most common in white, diamonds are also found in yellow and pink and more rarely in red, blue and green.

Diamonds are the emblem of love and fearlessness and also the symbol of purity. Thus they are the traditional stones for engagement rings. The left hand is related to the heart, so a diamond worn on the third finger of your left hand offers protection and love.

· 134 · *Friends for Life*

Buy – or better still get someone else to buy for you – the best diamonds you can afford. Bear in mind that in the upper echelons of diamond purity degrees of quality are only discernible to the experts, and then only with a super-powerful

*'The diamond is the common denominator of jew-
ellery.'*

—Nicola Bulgari

magnifying lens. But – and the same goes for men – don't settle for a diamond with obvious flaws.

If you want to know if a diamond is real or not, scratch it
against some glass. If it is real, it will cut it. Try this at the very
corner of a bathroom mirror, not anywhere a dirty great
scratch will matter.

The diamond will always be a signifier of wealth and class.
That is why it is a style classic. White diamonds go with everything, but they sparkle best when they are set in
platinum. Platinum is also a lighter metal than gold, thus
the obvious choice for tiaras.

Things a Woman Should Know About Style

If you are having a solitaire diamond engagement ring hold out for at least a carat. Remember when choosing an engagement ring that you will wear it for the rest of your life. Don't pick anything overly fashionable. Classic with a modern twist is good. Above all your ring should suit your personality.

One of the best – and worst – moments of a woman's life must be when that little black box is presented to her. Elation mixed with terror that you won't like the ring. Pray that your fiancé has good taste and if you don't like it saying so is better than keeping quiet. It will only surface in an argument down the line somewhere.

Different stones suit different occasions, outfits and moods. But diamonds will take you anywhere. Wear subtle diamond studs for day, long drop earrings and a line-bracelet at night. Start saving now, girls!

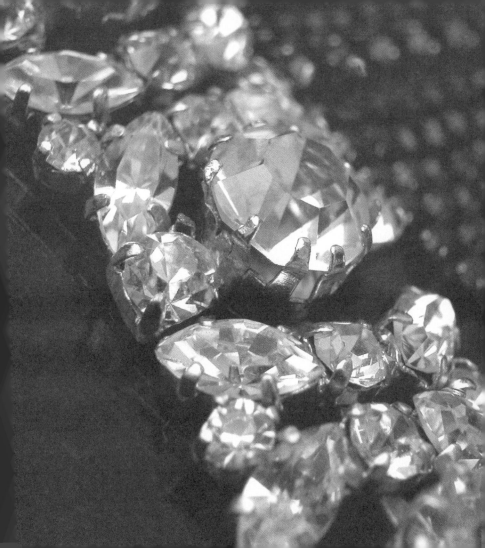

Heaven Scent

Putting on your diamonds and spraying yourself with scent are the completing acts of the stylish appearance.

A not unsurprising comment from the woman who set a precedent for profit by launching her infamous No. 5, the most famous perfume in the world.

Every woman searches for the olfactory Holy Grail that is a signature scent, only to be thwarted once again with a whiff of Issey Miyake on yet another woman. There is nothing more annoying than smelling your perfume on another woman. Except perhaps smelling it on a man. Beware of unisex fragrances; when you dress up for an evening you want to smell feminine and not the same as the maitre d'. That said, for daywear, the classic unisex cologne Acqua di Parma has a fresh, lemony charm perfect for lunching in Tuscan gardens. Fortunately perfume reacts differently on every individual's skin. So you won't smell exactly the same.

The chances of finding a perfume unique to you are non-existent. Unless you pay an expert 'nose' five hundred pounds to blend your own personal scent, like the woman who went with her fiancé to have a scent blended for her wedding night. At least you will be sure he likes it.

If your boyfriend says he doesn't like your perfume, stop wearing it immediately. If you find out your perfume is the same as his ex-girlfriend's stop wearing it even faster. Particularly if he says he does like it.

Be very, very suspicious if your boyfriend buys you the same perfume his ex wore. By the same token no matter how much you love your ex's cologne, don't buy it for anyone new.

Things a Woman Should Know About Style

If you are travelling away from someone you love spray their scent on a card and put it in your luggage. A sentimental arrival is guaranteed.

When choosing a perfume spray the tester on each wrist and let it settle for at least an hour before making your decision. Newly sprayed perfume smells of nothing but alcohol. The alcohol content of perfume makes it a very useful emergency pimple-blitzer if you are travelling.

The best place to find an exclusive scent is in an off-the-beaten track toiletries store in France, with its own cheap blend of toilet water. For extra cachet tell everyone it is very exclusive and not available in this country. This trick with local colognes doesn't work quite so well in Spain or Italy. Not unless you

'No elegance is possible without perfume.'

— Coco Chanel

want to smell like a teenage boy's bathroom the night he thinks he's going to lose his virginity.

When buying toilet water be discerning in your choice of flowers. Rosewater smells of the faded grandeur of old actresses; lavender smells of your granny.

Perfume makes money for struggling fashion houses. It is the fastest way to make money off a designer brand as anyone can buy into a lifestyle with a bottle of scent. Few new perfumes on the market endure like the classics. Chanel No.5 or anything created by Guerlain before 1930 are your safest bets.

Buy your perfume in a luxurious perfume hall in an exclusive department store and you could pay double for the shopping experience. Buy perfume in Superdrug. It all smells the same.

Like foodstuffs and medicines, perfume does have a sell-by date. A bottle of perfume once opened will not last more than six months. At least not to a nose that knows.

Painting by Numbers

Remember your teenage attempts at make-up? Electric blue mascara, blusher that couldn't decide if it went from the top of your ear to your chin, or straight across from lobe to lips, and orange foundation that stopped in a definite line beneath your chin. These are the mistakes that teach us what good make-up should look like. Especially when we see the photos.

Make-up should enhance, not camouflage. The natural look is enduringly chic.

Painting by Numbers

Make-up has as many trends as any other fashion so try to ignore the retro vogue for pastel eyeshadows in apricot and lime, and treble-thickness false eyelashes. A decent thickening mascara will stand you in far better stead than false eyelashes will any day.

Wear black mascara for night and dark brown mascara for day. Wear coloured mascara if you are going to a Biba revival party and nowhere else. There is nothing so pointless as clear mascara. It is a mystery why anyone bothered to invent it.

Dyeing your eyelashes works a treat if you are lazy.

'Before she allows the world to judge her face, a woman is entitled to create it.'

— Kennedy Fraser

Things a Woman Should Know About Style

Foundation should match the tone of the skin on your face. Test it on the side of your face between lower cheek and chin. Don't test it on your hand. Hold up your hand to your face. Is it the same colour? No! Face the fact that you might need a pale shade for winter and a darker one for summer. In between times mix them up together.

Black women take your cue from Iman and her inspiring range of make-up for dark skins.

Use foundation sparingly, mixing it with a moisturiser if it is lumpy.

Foundation is an excellent sunblock. As the improbably young-looking Ms Joan Collins always claimed, wear it every day and you won't get wrinkles.

If foundation is separating in the pot shake it. If it is still separating throw it out.

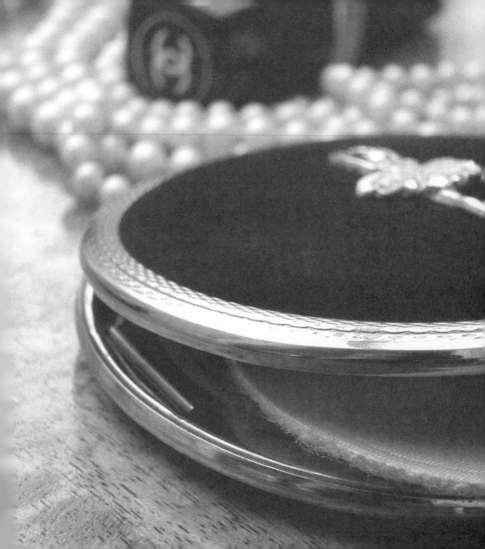

Things a Woman Should Know About Style

If you buy nothing else, buy Touche Eclat, the miracle concealer stick from Yves St Laurent, and say goodbye to dark eyes. Until you wake up in the morning at least.

Mascara and evenly toned skin are all you need to help your classic beauty along, with a lick of subtle lipstick on occasion.

A woman only needs two lipsticks: almost nude for day and darkish red for night. I'm sure I don't need to explain what kind of signals fire-engine red lipstick sends out. Or frosted pink for that matter.

The beauty industry is big business. It is all very well being able to dress the part but true style comes from within and if the body you inhabit is neglected you won't feel good, so you won't look good.

Do as the French do and allocate yourself a monthly beauty budget. Then start paying attention to parts of your body you may have forgotten existed.

Feet are the most neglected part of the body. Stuffed into ill-fitting shoes and forced to carry great weight, it is no wonder feet end up in such a state. No one likes to discover, on the first day of an expensive beach holiday, a lizard-like creature of white and puckered flesh, horned yellow talons clawing at new sandals. It doesn't have to be this way. Feet can be butter-soft, sweet smelling and prettily painted the colour of roses. Maintenance can be done at home, but for serious transformation go to a beauty salon and get a pedicure.

Pedicures are good for the sole. Sorry!

It takes regular pedicures to have truly beautiful feet. Pedicures in winter are especially gratifying, but walking out in the pour-

'In the factory we make cosmetics; in the store we sell hope.'

— Charles Revson (founder of Revlon)

ing rain with flip-flops on is not. But if you don't wear flip flops, the insides of your socks will resemble the make-up department of ER. There is a trick that involves a droplet of oil on each painted nail and wrapping your toes in clingfilm before putting your shoes back on, but it doesn't always work. Chances are that after slipping about in your shoes all the way home, crinkling as you walk, you will still take off your socks to a blood-bath.

Be really indulgent and take a taxi home in bare feet.

Manicures are only good for women who don't do the washing up. Manicures are hugely frustrating because you can't do anything with your hand for an hour after having one. For example, undo your buttons to go to the loo. If having a manicure, go to the loo beforehand and take your card out of your wallet ready to pay.

To resurrect your hands after too much washing up, smear them with Vaseline and wrap them in gloves overnight.

Potentially messy but worth it when you wake up with baby-soft skin.

Say 'Yes' to facials, 'No' to face-lifts. What sane person would willingly put themselves through the pain and risk of an unnecessary operation? Tie your hair in a super-tight pony-tail for the same effect. As for Botox, please! Knowingly injecting yourself with botulism combined with the embarrassment of looking like a Barbie doll because you've lost the ability to express yourself facially.

Try a facial workout. A grimace a day keeps the wrinkles at bay.

Mind Over Matter

Smiling uses twice as many facial muscles as frowning and saves those ugly dents between the eyes. But beware of crows feet: you can't win.

Things a Woman Should Know About Style

'Mind rules the body, and if, with the practice of these exercises, the thought is held that you are drawing to yourselves the life force, you will actually draw it.'

— Elinor Glyn, *The Wrinkle Book*

Don't smoke. It will age you, then kill you. Ignore the fact that smoking still looks cool on certain stick-thin attitudinal models. Get someone to tell you how stupid you look smoking. It is the fastest way to give up.

Don't neglect your body in favour of your face. Or vice versa. Plump women often only see themselves from the neck up, preferring to ignore their more voluptuous regions. But thin women only see themselves from the neck down, choosing not to see that their face has thinned to scrawn.

Excess bodily hair is not stylish. Depilate. It is a myth that shaving makes hair grow back faster than waxing.

But re-growth can be uncomfortable in certain sensitive areas.

Know your waxes: the Brazilian: a Mohican; the Hollywood: smooth and naked as a newborn. Rather too *Lolita* to be tasteful.

A bikini line should be just that – the line where your bikini ends. Tell me someone you know who wears a bikini an inch wide?

Waxing legs takes less regular maintenance but abandon it if you are spending more time covering up regrowth than you are showing off newly waxed legs.

Exfoliation works miracles at stopping in-growing hairs.

Unfortunately some women are born hairy and some women aren't. Life's not fair.

Getting a tan makes everyone's legs look better. A light tan is much better than a dark one. Sitting in the sun may make you feel better but there is nothing worse than looking like a leathery crocodile-skin handbag. Coco Chanel always sported a deep tan because it was fashionable then to turn a dark mahogany. Look at a picture of Chanel in old age and her deeply etched lines speak for themselves. Today we know better. Fake it.

Alternatively, make a point of protecting your pale and interesting skin.

Until the early part of the twentieth century pale skin was seen as a sign of good breeding. But in the 1920s and '30s a suntan became fashionable as a symbol of wealth. It meant you could afford to travel abroad.

Package Deal

Tan or no tan, holidays are often a minefield of style disasters. The most stylish of women have their style radars short circuited by the scanners at the airport and think nothing of appearing on the beach in a towelling Mickey Mouse shorts and t-shirt set. Diana, Princess of Wales was a case in point, photographed on a private holiday in a kind of jump-suit version of the above.

It is tempting to abandon all your cares when you go away, including what you look like. But if you want to remain stylish in the sun, beach holidays are not the place for wearing any ten-year-old terry towelling shorts you happen to find at the back of your wardrobe. Nor is it acceptable to slip into your boyfriend's old boxers and vest: the cast of *Friends* may think they get away with it, but you won't.

Think Joan Collins, Katharine Hepburn or Princess Margaret: baggy, mannish white linen trousers and shirts, the odd brightly coloured caftan and a huge floppy straw hat to be worn with over-sized sunglasses. If you have Jackie Onassis' s figure throw in a Pucci dress. But don't risk all those pink and yellow swirls if you are over a size ten.

Get a floppy hat that folds up so you spare yourself the embarrassment of carrying it in rainy England. Don't buy a straw hat in any colour other than natural. Especially not pink. Black is tempting but will quickly make your head feel hotter than the lobster thrown into the boiling pot at your local seafood restaurant.

We all know it, but remember it: black absorbs the heat, white reflects it.

It is easy to forget how hot thin-seeming clothes can be, when in England we consider it a heatwave when the temperature reaches twenty degrees. Be honest about the cool-factor of your clothes in thirty-degree heat.

Don't get over-excited when it gets hot in this country. Particularly don't rush up to your nearest inner-city patch of grass and lie sprawled and pink-skinned in your bikini.

Linen – even black – feels cool, but is hell to keep looking good. Take a travel iron. Accept it will crease the moment you put it on. If you want to look good when you arrive, never wear linen on an aeroplane. Linen pyjama bottoms work just as well as trousers for a casual beach look and they're half the price. Plus the drawstring is very handy for extra holiday dining.

Things a Woman Should Know About Style

Packing linen in dry-cleaning bags will help keep it crease-free in your suitcase. In fact packing all your delicate fabrics such as silk in dry cleaning bags is a good idea. Your dry cleaner will give you some if you ask. Or you could always just have it all dry-cleaned every time you get back from a holiday and leave it in the bags. Alternatively use tissue paper.

Pack trousers or jeans rolled into a sausage shape, rather than folded, to avoid creasing.

Buy one of those brilliant dresses from Ghost that scrunch up into a ball and still look fantastic when you put them on at the other end. That's if you like the scrunched-dress look.

Squeeze knickers and socks into your shoes (not smelly old trainers) and put them at the bottom of your case. The stuffing will help to keep the shape of the shoes so you don't end up flattening your favourite pair of heels into a pair of espadrilles.

Accept the fact that you are always going to take five pairs of shoes but only wear one.

Avoid chunky sweaters. They take up too much space and the Michelin Man look is never flattering. Of course, if you are camping in Wales, do take a chunky sweater. And leave all those shoes behind, along with your vanity. There are times that style just has to go out of the window.

Capsule beach wardrobe: linen drawstring trousers; smart cotton trousers; selection of linen shirts; a crisp white t-shirt for every day you are away (forget washing, you're on holiday); movie-star kaftan; hat; selection of bikinis and swimming costumes; shoes and sandals.

Capsule city-break wardrobe: smart black trousers; white shirt for every day you are away; black sweater; selection of Hermes-style scarves; evening dress; flat shoes and heels. For work-trips just add a suit.

Things a Woman Should Know About Style

Don't waste space with full-sized bottles of shampoo, etc. Buy travel size bottles.

Remember that virtually everything can be bought at the airport. Your pre-trip mantra: tickets, credit card, passport.

Buy clever luggage. Bags that fold out into double the size are invaluable for sneaking back holiday purchases. Suitcases on wheels are essential unless you are driving door-to-door.

Not Waving but Drowning

The big dilemma: swimming costume or bikini? Be honest with yourself, do you have the physique of Victoria Beckham or Queen Victoria? Remember that you won't have the advantage of Queen Victoria's fully-dressed bathing ensemble nor her personal beach hut on wheels that allowed her to slip into the sea from a private changing room wheeled to the water's edge.

Only skinny girls with flat tummies and smooth rounded hips look good in string bikinis. Women with normal-sized chests need more than two tiny triangles of fabric on a bit of string to protect their modesty. An underwired, boned, wet-suit thick, black lycra swimming costume, for example. Interestingly, women of all sizes look good in wet-suits. Not that I'd advise dipping into the hotel pool in one.

Don't buy swimming costumes with padded cups. Soggy wads of fabric make for a misshapen bosom.

Buying a larger size in bikini bottoms is a good thing in that it stops that ugly bulge around the hips, but beware that when water-logged a cotton lycra bikini will stretch into a saggy and shapeless bit of old cloth.

Much swimwear is not designed for swimming. Be extra careful when diving into swimming pools. Your bikini bottoms (or top) may not be travelling on the same trajectory as you are. Worth checking they haven't slipped down to your knees

Things a Woman Should Know About Style

before surfacing triumphant from your perfect swallow dive. Buy a classic Speedo one-piece for getting wet and a stylish designer bikini that must on all accounts remain dry.

We've had the dry-clean only bathmat, so I'm sure it's only a matter of time before we encounter the dry-clean only bikini.

Reasonably high-cut costumes look better on almost everyone, even if you are curvy. They make legs look longer and waists look slimmer.

Swimming costumes with those retro '30s frills round the bottom are fine for six-year olds but rather fey for grown women. Particularly ones with polka dots.

Sarongs are useful for covering bottoms but wonderful, flamboyant kaftans are the only thing for true beach glamour. Particularly when worn lying by the pool of an expensive hotel, having a pedicure and sipping a cocktail.

Kaftans are best worn in Barbados or the Bahamas or lounging by the pool at a Beverly Hills hotel. They cover everything and still look stylish so you can eat lunch to your heart's content. Wear your hair tied casually back with a scarf, or if you want the full look wrap it all up in a turban. Accessorise with perfectly painted toes and real jewellery.

We all have fantasies when we stride through the airport that we are another person, with another, more glamorous life. So dress the part and you might find yourself ushered into the first class lounge or, better still, upgraded. Rumour has it that upgrades are determined by the look of the passenger. Look expensive. Wear sunglasses on your head, hook your handbag into the crook of your arm and assume an expression of nonchalance. Only do this in airports or designer boutiques. Nowhere else will you be taken seriously.

Things a Woman Should Know About Style

Luggage Says Everything

Louis Vuitton: Rock star's wife or 'It' girl. Don't even bother if you have only one bag; it is too humiliating to be looked down upon by those with the matching trunk set.

Mulberry: Says can't afford Louis Vuitton but think it is terribly vulgar anyway. Much rather have understated country-house elegance.

Prada: Italian 'It' boys.

Samsonite: Business trips.

Try to resist the personalised elastic to help you identify your suitcase on the baggage re-claim conveyor belt. Ok, so it's really ly useful.

Airports are just one of the places of anonymity and possibility that tempt us to believe we are someone other than we really are. I am sure that airlines are in cahoots with retailers in demanding such long check-in times. The combined effect of exhilaration about going on holiday and being trapped in a glossy duty-free shopping mall for two hours is potentially bankrupting.

A similar, yet far more dangerous threat to the bank balance is the designer boutique.

The Great Escape

Shopping is all about buying into a lifestyle. This is particularly true of clothes.

A designer coat is cheaper than a sports car.

Designer clothes are marketed to us as badges of the perfect life. It is no accident that designers are increasingly selling home products, bath products and *objets d'art*, lulling us into spending more money in the smart restaurants and coffee bars in their stores.

Beware of lunching in Nicole Farhi's restaurants. The food is excellent, but allowing oneself a glass of wine within staggering distance of the new autumn/winter collection is ill-advised.

Does buying designer buy you style? Sometimes but certainly not always. You are probably buying marginally better fabric and slightly more of it. But your dress, suit, coat is still machine-manufactured and, these days, unlikely to be finished by hand. You are paying for a label, for a name and for what that represents. Ostensibly you are also paying for design expertise.

A designer's mainline collection is where you will find genuinely innovative design, timeless classics and the finest fabrics. It is more expensive to buy Giorgio Armani than Emporio, but you are getting more 'designer'. Arguably designer diffusion lines are just a marketeer's dream: a way of cashing in on a brand without laying out the overheads. This is where you really pay for the label, perhaps not for the quality of the clothes.

Things a Woman Should Know About Style

You get good and bad clothes in every shop, designer or high street. Keep your wits about you and try to be objective.

Be wary of bewitching sales assistants' 'Come here, my pretty, and buy this dress.' This sales ploy is seductive: 'You too can be like me if you buy this dress (cackle, cackle)…' – you get the idea.

Worse still is the intimidation factor: skinny, snooty sales assistants scanning you from head to toe, making you feel like an amateur hand-thrown pot in a fine china shop, lumpy and

'A good many women who buy new clothes are afflicted by the delusions that they will thereby change their state of mind, the attitude of their companions and their lives.'

— Kennedy Fraser

coarse next to thin porcelain-skinned beauties. A sneer and a subtly arched eyebrow are all it takes to have you slinking back out of the door.

Bewitched

Beware the seduction of new clothes. All clothes are appealing when they do not belong to you. It is the possibility of something new that could turn you in to a new person that is so seductive, not the garment itself.

Similarly, being surrounded by brightly coloured or a particular style of clothes makes your classic black outfit seem instantly drab and unfashionable. Rather than immediately buying a pair of lilac hipsters, walk out onto the street, or into a store with plenty of black in it, and see if you still feel dowdy.

Shop in stores that are your style. If you are classic, shop in a store that carries suits, black trousers and elegant camel twinsets. Not one that tempts you with the promise of re-inventing yourself in fuschia pink PVC. Be strong.

Supermodel In the Mirror Syndrome: the slit-to-the-navel dress you are wearing may look great on Helena Christensen but does it really look good on you? Look in the mirror and see yourself. Can you really get away without wearing a bra?

By the same token, if friends, sales assistants and the hopeful voice inside your head are telling you a dress looks fantastic, believe it! This is no time to be self-deprecating.

Hype: just because everyone else is buying that must-have item, you don't have to. Sales assistants will tell you it has been flying out of the door, that they only have one left in your size, etc. Don't believe them. That said, if you find a truly superb outfit, that fits like a glove, is a little expensive but not absurdly so, buy it! Grasp sartorial gems when you see them and never, ever wait for the sale.

Sales Tactics

Sales shopping is a whole different ballgame. It must be the hunting instinct, but like dogs fighting to get the last scrap of meat, women turn into savages at the mention of a sale. Dale Winton would be proud of the assault a normally sane woman can make on her favourite store at sale time.

Clothes you would not have given a second glance at full price suddenly become desperately desirable when they go on sale, even more so when other women are just as desperate as you are. Just as your dull boyfriend becomes an Adonis when another woman looks at him, fighting the blond in the corner for a pair of orange satin-Lycra disco trousers becomes a matter of life or death. The golden rule of sales shopping is to buy only what you would have considered buying at full price. Don't just buy because it's cheap.

There is a reason clothes are on sale: not enough people wanted to buy them at full price. Think about it.

Sale clothes are more likely to be fashion pieces than classic pieces. Classic pieces – black trousers and suits, for example – are considered part of many stores' core collections that never go on sale.

Watch out for stores trying to off-load years-old stock at sale time.

There are only two days of the sales worth going to: the first and the last. On the first, the choicest items will fly out of the door. As the reductions aren't huge at the beginning, stick to classics you'll wear for more than one season. Wait until that red-leather catsuit is half-price before you give in, and then only if you genuinely love it. If you see something good on the first day of the sale don't be tempted to wait for it to be reduced further. If you think it's a bargain so will someone else and they'll buy it first. This is particularly true of shoes where popular sizes sell out fast.

Reductions tend to go in three waves: twenty to thirty percent off, fifty percent off and 'crazy prices, last day of sale' seventy percent off. That is why it's worth going on the last day too.

The couple of days before the sales start you might find pen-cilled numbers on the back of garments, or find that clothes are shifted into sections. This is the shop getting ready, so pay heed and you could have a head start. If you are really lucky, some stores have computer systems that take so long to update with sales prices they show up before the sale officially starts. Worth a try the day before.

Things a Woman Should Know About Style

Sales often mean chaos for sales staff. If something is wrongly priced by them you are within your rights to ask to pay that price. They don't have to sell it to you, they can withdraw it, but a retailer can't insist you pay a higher price.

Sales are brilliant times to pick up classic designer clothes at good prices but you need to put your time in. Go everywhere, keep your head, don't panic buy and be honest about whether clothes fit, look good, or are going to go out of fashion fast.

Try not to let your genuine bargains be outweighed by your mistakes. Otherwise you might as well have bought the one decent outfit – amongst the glitter, colour and too-small fantasy-me clothes – for full price.

Sales are good for buying clothes you have to buy: suits for work, for example.

A Uniform Workforce

It is a perverse trick of psychology that having to wear suits for work immediately makes you want to throw on the nearest pair of jeans and trainers. Typically, as soon as 'dress-down' policies at work became ubiquitous, suits came back into fashion with a vengeance.

Many companies thought they'd hit the nail on the head with a dress-down workwear ethic. However, after legions of accountants alarmed their directors by dressing like yachties, there has been a backlash. On the whole, a policy of treading the middle line is best; after all there is nothing so embarrassing as having to face your boss and his most important client wearing clothes that make you look like a teenager.

Fact: you are more likely to look stylish – and professional – if you are wearing a suit.

The essential formal working wardrobe: three-piece suits: jacket, trousers and skirt; black and beige stretch trousers; pencil skirts and tidy sweaters; fitted shirts and heavy white cotton t-shirts; good belts; fine leather flat shoes and heels you can walk in for power meetings; the most expensive and capacious handbag you can afford.

The essential dressed-down working wardrobe: the same as for formal work-wear bar the jacket of your suits (you can keep this on the back of your chair for meeting emergencies). If you can get away with it add a pressed pair of dark blue jeans that flatter you. When trying on jeans, be honest with yourself.

Choose trouser suits or 1940s-style, nipped in at the waist, 'Miss Moneypenny' suits. Avoid the dreaded 'inverted triangle' that typified the 1980s.

Trouser suits are fantastic. They can be simple and stylish (Lady Helen Taylor), boyish and independent (Katharine Hepburn) or lean and mean (Marlene Dietrich). Wear them to meetings, parties, premieres and dinners. You'll never have to get your legs waxed or buy another pair of tights again. Wear them with heels for maximum woman-power, with flats for suburban chic and funky Prada 'trainers' (keep them black and leather) for a fashion statement.

Unless you work in media industries where jeans are as much a uniform as pinstripe is in the city, leave your very casual clothes for the weekend.

If you are trying to be stylish... leave your trainers at home.

It is hard to feel stylish at work as at least half the challenge of exuding style is feeling it. And let's face it, drowning under a mountain of emails, with your boss shouting at you to meet a deadline is hardly conducive to feeling like an icon of style. Fantasy has a lot to do with it so, once you've got the clothes right, pretending to be your favourite film star/model/Euro-royal will work wonders on your attitude.

Classic film-star glamour from the 'good ole studio days' is what you are after. Films to watch for style tips: *Breakfast at Tiffany's*, *Casablanca*, anything from the 1930s.

Ultimate (and varied) classic style icons to aspire to: Jackie Onassis, Grace Kelly, Audrey Hepburn, Katharine Hepburn, Marilyn Monroe, Elizabeth Taylor (in her girlish youth not elderly eccentricity), Ingrid Bergman, etc. The list of stylish actresses of the 1930s, '40s, and '50s is endless.

It is safer to stick to stars of the past, but if you are looking for a modern day role model think along the lines of Lady Helen Taylor (of course it helps if you are an ambassador for

Armani), Nicole Kidman or Halle Berry. Be careful to emulate a celebrity with real style. Never copy a woman who has had breast implants.

Remember that style comes from within.

Money Can't Buy
You...

Wearing the right clothes is not enough. Sorry. The way you carry yourself and the way you behave are just as important. Time to start acting like a lady. You owe it to yourself.

Wearing different clothes makes you feel and act differently. Put on a pair of stupidly high heels to walk with an exaggerated wiggle, a perfectly tailored suit or fitted dress to feel like you have the body of a supermodel, or a pair of wide, baggy sailor pants and white pumps to feel at home on a croquet lawn or in the *Great Gatsby*.

'Style is not something applied. It is something inherent, something that permeates... It is not a dress.'

— Wallace Stevens

Accessorise high heels and dresses with champagne, linen trousers and shirts or summer frocks with Pimms, everything else with fine wine in crystal glasses.

Carry yourself well. Walk tall and proud. Think of all those pictures of debutantes with piles of books on their heads. Your back will thank you in the long run. As will your clothes.

It has traditionally been deemed terribly bad manners for a woman to cross her legs at the knee. Well-brought up young gals cross at the ankle. Take the Queen as your example.

Things a Woman Should Know About Style

*'There are three things a woman ought to look:
straight as a dart, supple as a snake and proud as a
tiger-lily.'*

— Elinor Glyn

Nothing looks good on a hunched and rounded body.

Few people are aware of what correct etiquette is anymore. Fewer still really care. Use your common sense and try not to offend anyone. And hold your knife and fork properly.

Handbag Science

In psycho-analysis the handbag can be read as a symbol of a woman's sense of self. Take heed of dreams about losing or forgetting your handbag. If this is true, the post-traumatic stress resulting from actually having your handbag stolen is too awful to contemplate.

'A handbag!'

— Lady Bracknell in Oscar Wilde,
The Importance of Being Earnest

Things a Woman Should Know About Style

Carry bags close to your chest on public transport and never, ever put your handbag down in a bar. In restaurants eat with your bag sitting on your lap or clamped between your legs. You may feel silly, but better silly than sorry. At parties leave your bag at home. Make your boyfriend carry your lipstick in his pocket.

Losing your handbag is traumatic but increasingly common. To minimise potential upset photocopy your address book, back up your mobile phone number list and don't keep your chequebook in the same bag as your credit card (though in practice this is nigh on impossible). Insure everything: phone, jewellery, watch, handbag itself. Check your policy – items lost or stolen out of the home aren't always automatically covered.

What you carry in your handbag says more about you than you think. Clear out those half-eaten chocolate bars and unpaid credit card bills

Women have one of two relationships with their handbags: monogamy or promiscuity. Try to be faithful, particularly to Italians of impeccable pedigree.

The 'Vaseline, Life in a Bag' exhibition of 2001 was held at Selfridges department store and celebrated fifty years of women's handbags. A survey carried out prior to exhibition painted an intriguing picture of twenty-first century woman. Condoms, contraceptive pills and donor cards spell responsibility; filofaxes, electronic organisers and laptops point to organised lives; but cigarettes – 21 percent of women surveyed carried them – and indigestion tablets far outweighed gym kits.

Half a century ago we weren't so different. A handbag might have contained a ration book and Players cigarettes, but the 1950s girl still carried a tube map, painkillers, stockings and make-up.

Things a Woman Should Know About Style

An all-purpose handbag should be as big and as expensive as you can afford. Don't buy designer rip-offs. So what if no-one else knows. You do. Don't waste your money on designer black nylon – put it towards saving for a decent leather bag.

Think of a bag as an investment. You want it to be stylish and value for money (it can be expensive and still be value for money if you use it for years).

The doyen of all handbags is the Hermes Kelly Bag, named after Grace Kelly used it to disguise her pregnancy before determined paparazzi. If you haven't got thousands of pounds or a year to spare on the waiting list, buy J. P. Tod's. Know an acceptable alternative when you see one.

The law of handbag desirability obeys an inverse ratio of price to size. The smaller and pricier the better. Known to ladies who lunch as the 'status bag'. Use your standard nylon holdall/backpack/briefcase during the day, then pull out your status bag for power-lunching or dates.

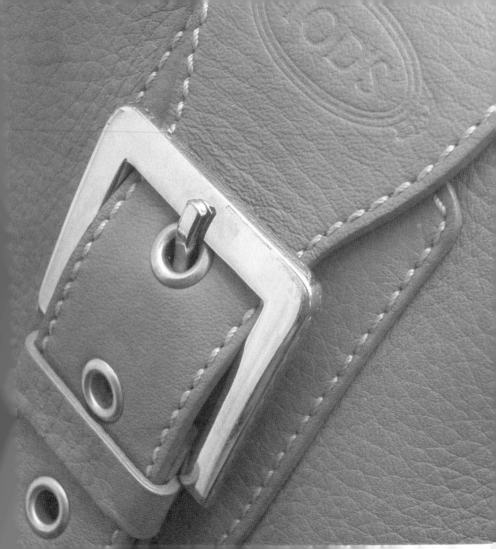

Things a Woman Should Know About Style

Be careful what status you are proclaiming. Your bag may be saying something about you that you would rather not hear:

Prada and Gucci: Footballers' wives.

Fendi: Try-hard fashion victim. Anything a member of the public can get their hands on is bound to be way out of date.

Louis Vuitton: Coloured, grained leather: jet-setting banker or CEO; traditional monogrammed: wannabe ladies-who-lunch; graffiti: gangsters' girlfriends.

Never, ever buy a 'graffiti bag'. Even the genuine ones look like fakes.

Forget about the label and concentrate on the quality. Buy genuinely beautiful Italian leather in Florentine markets. Stick your nose in the air and say, 'What do you mean you've never heard of...'

You will always need more than one handbag. In fact you can justify an almost limitless number. Like shoes, handbags are something a girl can always do with more of.

Necessary handbags: a large black for winter; tan for summer; leather tote-bag; a range of smaller clutch, evening and lunchtime bags; a woven tote in stylish 'naturals' for the beach, summer holidays, etc.

When you really hit the big time you'll want bags to match all your shoes. Ah well, a girl can dream can't she?

Get into the backpack, the over-the-shoulder and the hand-held tote debate at your peril. It is pretty conclusive: backpacks are far better for your back and posture, but far worse for your style credibility. No matter how hard Prada, Louis Vuitton et al try to convince us otherwise, backpacks make clothes look terrible. Hand-held totes are marginally better for posture, but only if you balance the other side of your body with an equally heavy bag. A good excuse to go shopping, I suppose.

Shoulder-bags should be light. A light handbag is an oxymoron. Women have been known to carry a good quarter of their bodyweight around with them daily. Think about it: purse, keys, mobile phone, filofax/organiser, book for reading on train, umbrella-gloves-sunglasses trio for unpredictable British weather, notebook and pen, child paraphernalia, bottle of water, emergency snack – the list is endless.

Take care of your bag: don't over-stuff it.

Hard leathers are more structured, so allow more stuffing in without complete loss of shape, but they scratch more easily and bulge less attractively. There are arguments that soft leathers are better as they get more pliable, rich and sensuous with wear. Soft leather bags will mould to the shape of their contents so don't carry spare shoes. Especially not stilettos. A razor-sharp heel in contact with a kid-skin bag doesn't bear thinking about. Another reason to wear shoes (NOT trainers!) to work.

Be careful where you put down your bag – not just because it might get stolen, it might get filthy. Buy pale leather bags at your peril. Camel is a better light alternative than cream.

If your bag suffers from exposure to car-fumes, park benches and taxi floors, give it the same treatment as you would your face: cleanse and moisturise with leather products. It is skin after all. All leather benefits from being looked after. Buy some Leather Food and feed away. Uncared for leather will dry out and crack. Just like uncared-for complexions.

Scotchguard pale leather shoes, bags and coats (and sofas, carpets, etc.).

Right On

Wearing leather is – aside from in a few vegan communes – acceptable worldwide. Wearing fur is fraught with danger and varies wildly as you cross international borders.

Fur coats are coveted in Europe – France, Italy and Spain in particular – but risqué in the UK and US. Unfortunately, fashion changes so fast it can be real on the catwalk one moment, fake the next. Safer not to, if you're worried. Fur-trim coats are easier to get away with. Buy them in Italy.

Fake fur is pretty convincing these days and on sight few people can tell the difference, which is good news whatever your politics. Touch a fake fur and you will know immediately, however. The purist would argue why wear something fake at all? Either wear real fur and stand by your decision or wear something else. If you are going to buy fur, buy mink.

Appease your conscience and buy only vintage furs. If you can bear the musty smell.

Unless you want people to think you are raving mad, avoid fox-fur stoles with the heads still intact. The same goes for ferrets.

Fur coats are unsuitable for women under forty years of age or five feet in height. Short round women in fur look like Mrs Tiggywinkle.

Fur hats – only in Russia.

Things a Woman Should Know About Style

Fur-lined gloves – essential if you have poor circulation.

It is not just fur coats that should last you a life-time. I'm assuming that if you are interested enough in clothes to be reading this book, you possess more than one winter coat that you replace when it wears out...

A Winter's Tale

Buy classic black cashmere or fine wool, crombie-style, three-quarter length, single breasted, with covered buttons, slightly fitted at the waist. Make sure the sleeves are long enough and watch out for over-padded shoulders.

Next buy a camel belted coat – same length, same fabric.

Full-length coats in wool are dated-looking, unless you are talking full-length, 'Oh my God, I've died and gone to heaven' sheepskin. Totally glamorous and horribly, deliciously expensive. If you ever get the opportunity to own one of these choose black or dark brown. Camel or beige are tempting but stupidly impractical and not at all flattering unless you are Elizabeth Hurley on a well-airbrushed day.

Sheepskin, leather and suede need specialist cleaning that can cost a lot of money, so be careful where you wear it. The softer the leather the more careful you need to be about brushing up against rough surfaces. One chip in a door-frame is all it takes.

For daywear, by all means wear a stylish, microfibre coat, but not if it calls itself an anorak.

The coat you are wearing should go with the style of whatever is underneath. Don't wear a puffa to a black-tie dinner. The same applies to lengths. Coats should be ideally the same length as the skirt beneath them.

Denim jackets worn under woollen coats might have looked

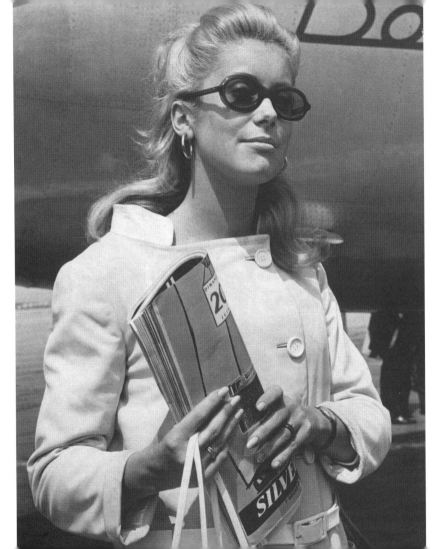

cool when you were a student, but anyone over thirty will look like they are trying way too hard. Denim jackets are risky per se, when it comes to achieving an image of classic style. Maybe a dark one, over black trousers on a weekend. Denim jackets with jeans only look good if a) they match perfectly and b) you are a nineteen-year-old supermodel.

Be glad you are not a model. Being judged by your looks is a nightmare most of us never really have to face. Try that on your self-esteem. Be pleased you don't have to look perfect every day and waking up with an enormous spot is an inconvenience and not a lost day's work.

The Last Word in...

After reading this book I hope you are convinced that looking good, dressing up and having fun with clothes is a pleasure no woman should deny herself. But I'm not advocating becoming one of those women imprisoned by her need to look perfect every second of her life. Chance would be a fine thing!

A sense of style is not about obsessing over the latest fashions... and finding your own style isn't as difficult as you might have thought.

Things a Woman Should Know About Style

'Fashion can make you ridiculous; style, which is yours to control individually, can make you attractive — a near siren.'

— Marianne Moore

Once you've found it, you will always know you've got it, even if you are dressed in your baggy old jeans and husband's shirt, cleaning the house on a Sunday. Of course there are certain times – ex-boyfriend's wedding, fortieth birthday party, job interview – when dressing to kill gives you the edge. And now you know how to tape your breasts into a slash-front, backless

'Style ain't nothing but keeping the same idea from beginning to end. Everybody got it.'

— August Wilson

frock, pick a dress that will have every man in the room drooling and walk in a pair of shoes that will give you four inches in height but four feet in confidence.

Style comes from the inside, so until you are happy in your own skin, you won't look good in anyone else's.

> *'Know, first, who you are; and then adorn yourself accordingly.'*
>
> — Epictetus

What you choose to wear says a lot about you... not all of it true.

Enjoy discovering your style... but don't get too neurotic or you'll turn into *one of those women.*

Things a Woman Should Know About Style

At the end of the day, you just take it all off again…

…and that's when you really know you're stylish.

'When I free my body from its clothes, from all their buttons, belts and laces, it seems to me that my soul takes a deeper, freer, breath.'

— August Strindberg